THE COOL IMPOSSIBLE

THE COOL IMPOSSIBLE

The Running Coach from *Born to Run* Shows How to Get the Most from Your Miles— and from Yourself

ERIC ORTON

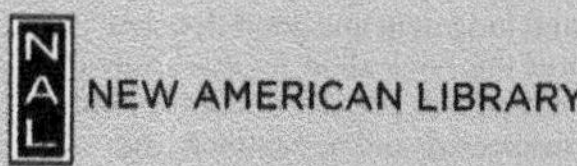

NEW AMERICAN LIBRARY

New American Library
Published by the Penguin Group
Penguin Group (USA) LLC, 375 Hudson Street,
New York, New York 10014

USA | Canada | UK | Ireland | Australia | New Zealand | India | South Africa | China
penguin.com
A Penguin Random House Company

Published by New American Library, a division of Penguin Group (USA) LLC. Previously published in a New American Library hardcover edition.

First New American Library Trade Paperback Printing, May 2014

NEW AMERICAN LIBRARY TRADE PAPERBACK ISBN: 978-0-451-41634-6

THE LIBRARY OF CONGRESS HAS CATALOGED THE HARDCOVER EDITION OF THIS TITLE AS FOLLOWS:
Orton, Eric.
The cool impossible: the running coach from born to run shows how to get the most from your miles and from yourself/Eric Orton.
p. cm.
ISBN 978-0-451-41633-9
1. Running-Training. I. Title.
GV1061.5.078 2013
796.42—dc23 2012050880

Printed in the United States of America

Set in Minion Pro
Designed by Pauline Neuwirth

PUBLISHER'S NOTE
While the author has made every effort to provide accurate telephone numbers, Internet addresses and other contact information at the time of publication, neither the publisher nor the author assumes any responsibility for errors, or for changes that occur after publication. Further, publisher does not have any control over and does not assume any responsibility for author or third-party Web sites or their content.

Every effort as been made to ensure that the information contained in this book is complete and accurate. However, neither the publisher nor the author is engaged in rendering professional advice or services to the individual reader. The ideas, procedures, and suggestions contained in this book are not intended as a substitute for consulting with your physician. All matters regarding your health require medical supervision. Neither the author nor the publisher shall be liable or responsible for any loss or damage allegedly arising from any information or suggestion in this book. The opinions expressed in this book represent the personal views of the author and not of the publisher.

Outdoor recreational activities are by their very nature potentially hazardous. All participants in such activities must assume the responsibility for their own actions and safety. If you have any health problems or medical conditions, consult with your physician before undertaking any outdoor activities. The information contained in this guide book cannot replace sound judgment and good decision making, which can help reduce risk exposure, nor does the scope of this book allow for disclosure of all the potential hazards and risks involved in such activities. Learn as much as possible about the outdoor recreational activities in which you participate, prepare for the unexpected, and be cautious. The reward will be a safer and more enjoyable experience.

To Angel:
Climb on through life, pumpkin!

To Michelle:
Because of you, my passion came to life and anything became possible!

ACKNOWLEDGMENTS

Where to begin but at the beginning: Thanks so much to my parents for their unconditional love and support and never asking, "Why?" Dad, thanks for teaching me that "can't never did anything."

To all of my athletes, this book was really written by you, and without our partnership, it would not have been possible. A big kudos in particular to Terry Hong (my Speedy Dot connector), Margot Watters, Jenn Sparks, Annie Putnam, George Putnam, and Keith Peters for your long-term commitment and trust in my training, and for so greatly influencing my Cool Impossible.

Thanks, coaches Nugent, Havens, and Schlageter for the life lessons you taught on the gridiron all those years ago. I'm still using them—often every day. And to all of my coaches—wow, there've been a lot of them over the years—who taught me the importance of fundamentals, technique, repetition, and perfect practice.

Paul Knutson, I appreciate your showing me the way—run in peace, my friend. Patrick Kelly, your five a.m. training wake-up calls are how Cool Impossibles are made. Thanks for all of our great training runs, swims, rides, and snowshoes.

Christopher McDougall, your relentless pursuit for truth is inspiring. Big thanks for your dedication and trust and never believing "you shouldn't" or "you are not meant to." Sawing logs forever!

Neal Bascomb, timing is everything. Thanks for being the race director for my Cool Impossible ultramarathon. Your direction and guidance really made this all possible, and there's no way I would have run that fast and well without you! And, man, your book *The Perfect Mile* really inspired.

Scott Waxman, my agent, thanks for being my coach down the literary trail, providing direction and quick solutions when things got steep and rocky. Your encouragement to follow my true voice gave me the confidence I needed as a rookie author.

Claire Zion, my editor, thanks for guiding this project with a sure hand and showing me the right path to the finish line.

Micah True, aka Caballo Blanco—you showed us all how to live the Cool Impossible. Run free. And thanks, Mas Locos everywhere, for keeping Caballo's dream alive.

And finally to you, my readers: Thanks for taking this journey with me. I wish you great success with your running and your own Cool Impossible. I would also like to ask for your help, to challenge and encourage you to be a part of my Cool Impossible by seeking out and helping beginning runners. See how many people you can inspire to start running. Share your knowledge with them. Offer to take them for runs on your easy recovery days. Let us create a world full of runners.

CONTENTS

FOREWORD xi

1. ME AND THE COOL IMPOSSIBLE 1
2. YOU IN GLORIOUS JACKSON HOLE 13
3. TRUE STRENGTH 27
4. PERFORMANCE RUNNING 85
5. STRATEGIC RUNNING FOUNDATION 117
6. EAT WELL, RUN WELL 181
7. PUTTING IT ALL TOGETHER 207
8. ATHLETICISM = AWARENESS 217
9. THE COOL IMPOSSIBLE 243

FOREWORD

by Christopher McDougall

IT'S EMBARRASSING, BUT it's taken me until now to really understand what Eric Orton has been telling me since the day we met. It's a classic case of missing the forest for the trees, except for me the forest was very strange and there was a naked woman running around in there, so you can understand how it could all get confusing.

I got to know the woman first. In the summer of 2005, a friend who'd served as a forest ranger invited me to join him and four of his pals on a three-day, fifty-mile trail-running trip through Idaho's River of No Return Wilderness. Our gear and food would be hauled by a mule packer, so all the six of us had to do was focus on running fifteen miles a day from campsite to campsite.

It was too sweet an offer to turn down, even though I wasn't much of a runner. Actually, I was close to being an *ex*-runner; I'd been laid up by a string of injuries over the previous few years, and three separate doctors had warned me that impact breakdowns were inevitable for six-foot-four 240-pounders like me. Ironically, I was writing for *Runner's World* at the time, so it wasn't as if I were lacking for injury-prevention and training advice. I'd tried every tip you'll find in a running magazine—stretching, cross-training, replacing my $150 shoes every four months with a fresh pair, heat-molded custom insoles, even icy-cold postrun soaks in a creek—but no matter what, it was only a matter of months before fiery twinges began shooting out from my knees, or heels, or hamstrings, or Achilles tendons.

Luckily, I was in the middle of a healthy streak when I got the Idaho invitation, so I said, "Sure, I'm in." On our first morning, I fell into stride behind a former ranger named Jenni Blake. She was as smooth over wind-fallen logs as water, just kissing the tree trunk with a tap of her shoe as she hurdled over and surged on, never breaking pace. Her full-body approach to running was a revelation; she flung her arms wide for balance on downhills, twisted her hips like a salsa dancer on sharp switchbacks, bent her knees deep when she hit a patch of scree and came churning right back out the other side. Her nimbleness and raw strength were so impressive, I was surprised to discover that for half her life, Jenni wasn't athletic at all.

"I really didn't know anything about the woods till I came to Idaho," Jenni told me when we stopped for a breather. "I was bulimic in college and had a terrible self-image, until I found myself out here."

She came as a summer volunteer, and was thrown right into the deep end: She was loaded up with a lumberjack saw, a Pulaski ax, and two weeks of freeze-dried food, and pointed toward the backcountry to go clear trails. She nearly buckled under the weight of the backpack, but she kept her doubts to herself and set off, alone, into the woods.

After a few days, Jenni was surprised to learn that the body she'd always hated was strong enough to swing an ax and muscle a downed lodgepole pine off the trail. She'd found it hard to hold back a sweaty smile as she stood atop Mosquito Ridge and looked down at the mile-high hill she'd just climbed. And when she wandered into the path of a marauding moose, she made another discovery: She was *fast*! The big brute burst out of the brush without warning, so before Jenni knew what she was doing, her legs were carrying her down the trail ahead of the lunging antlers. By the time the moose gave up, Jenni felt terrified, exhausted . . . and fantastic.

After that, she couldn't wait to roll out of her tent at daybreak. She'd pull on sneakers and nothing else, then set off for long runs through the woods, the rising sun warming her naked body. "I'd be out here for weeks at a time by myself," Jenni explained. "No one could see me, so I'd just go and go and go. It was the most fantastic feeling you can imagine." She didn't need a watch or a route; she judged her speed by the tickle of wind on her skin, and kept racing along the pine-needled trails until her legs and lungs begged her to head back to camp. Jenni paid for her nude morning miles later in the day, when her thighs got wobbly during long hikes, but her runs only got longer; this new romance with her body was too exciting to quit.

Jenni has been running wild ever since. She and her best pal, Nancy Hatfield, are leaders of an unstoppable all-gal running gang; after a snowstorm, they'll hit the roads around their hometown of McCall, Idaho, before the plows, and break their own trails through the snowdrifts.

"Winter running is the best!" chimed in Nancy, who was with us for the trek. Like Jenni, Nancy is a living rebuttal to the notion that twenty years of daily miles are a crippler; at forty-seven, she still runs the way a mermaid swims, with her brown hair cascading down her back, her legs swift yet languid, and even a sea blue belly ring winking in her navel.

But for me, that running vacation turned out to be a crippler. When I winced my way down the final downhill leg at the end of the third day, I could barely walk. My heels were stinging and both Achilles tendons were inflamed. I hobbled into the creek and sat there, simmering and wondering what was wrong with me. How come two middle-aged women could rip through mile after mile, year after year, on dirt and snow and tarmac, while I couldn't go more than a few months without coming apart?

The answer was right in front of my eyes, of course. Right there in the forest. I just didn't know what I was looking for.

A few weeks after my Idaho debacle, I was given an assignment by *Men's Journal* magazine to interview an adventure-sport coach based in Jackson Hole, Wyoming. My editor was intrigued, because Eric's specialty was tearing endurance sports down to their integral movements and finding transferable skills. Eric would study rock climbing to find shoulder techniques for kayakers, and apply Nordic skiing's smooth propulsion to mountain biking.

What Eric is really looking for, I discovered after I met up with him in Denver, are basic engineering principles; he's convinced that the next great advance in fitness will come not from training or technology, but technique: The athlete who avoids injury will be the one who leaves the competition behind. Curiously, no fitness activity offered more room for improvement than running. As the world's oldest and most popular sport, you'd think we'd have perfected it by now, but running has become a high-risk enterprise. More than 50 percent of all runners are injured every year, and always have been since running injury data was first collected in the 1970s—meaning I was the rule, not the exception. If someone could eliminate that risk factor, tremendous leaps forward were possible not just in performance, but in participation. Imagine the millions of people who wanted to run but were prevented by injuries, and the millions of others who'd heard the stories of ruined knees and were afraid to even try, all of them now free from pain and fear.

But for Eric, the only mystery was why it was so mysterious: Change what your body does, and you'll change what happens to your body. If you're getting injured from running, he believes, the next step is logical: You have to change the way you run.

"Everyone thinks they know how to run, but it's really as nuanced as any other activity," Eric told me. "Ask most people and they'll say, 'People just run the way they run.' That's ridiculous. Does everyone just swim the way they swim?" For every other sport, lessons are fundamental; you don't go out and start slashing away with a golf club or sliding down a mountain on skis until someone takes you through the steps and teaches you proper form. If not, inefficiency is guaranteed and injury is inevitable.

"Running is the same way," Eric explained. "Learn it wrong, and you'll never know how good it can feel."

Wait; why had I never heard this before? Once he spelled it out, it seemed painfully obvious. *Of course* there had to be a right and a wrong way to run. There's a better and worse way to perform every biomechanical motion on earth, from throwing a ball to eating with chopsticks.

Why would running be the only activity on the planet that was free from the laws of physics? But I'd never heard this line of thought before. All I ever read about in running magazines was what to buy—motion-controlling shoes, orthotics, compression socks—not what to *do*.

And then Eric added something that, to my big man's ears, was strange, beautiful music.

"Everyone is built for running."

For years, I'd been told just the opposite: Doctors and physical therapists kept telling me that running is bad for the body, especially bodies built on the same specs as Shrek's. And I believed it, because I felt the proof in my aching Achilles. Eric then offered to back up his bravado: He volunteered to coach me by e-mail and transform me from an ailing ex-runner into not just a marathoner, but an ultramarathoner. In nine months, he promised, I'd be able to handle a fifty-mile race through the Copper Canyon of Mexico with the legendary Tarahumara Indians.

Naturally, I was enticed, but I'd also been enticed by the Idaho trip, and I'd seen how that turned out. I'd spent three days covering fifty miles, and I finished it plopped in a creek and vowing I'd never do anything that stupid again. Now Eric was not only proposing I run fifty miles in a single day, but also ramp up my mileage way faster than the 10-percent-per-week rule that the running magazines always preach. There was no way I'd get to the race, I thought; the workouts would finish me off first.

"Every time I up my miles," I replied, "I break down."

"You won't this time."

"Should I get the orthotics?"

"Forget the orthotics."

I was still dubious, but Eric's absolute confidence was winning me over. "I should probably cut weight first to make it easier on my legs."

"Your diet will change all by itself. Wait and see."

"How about yoga? That'll help, yeah?"

"Forget yoga and stretching. Muscle tightness is not solved by stretching."

I was already liking the sound of this. No diet, no yoga, no orthotics. I was wavering.

"You really think I can do this?"

"Here's the truth," Eric said. "You've got zero margin of error. But you can do it."

Lost as I was in my own concerns about the challenge, I never really considered the challenge that was facing Eric. Not only did he have to rehabilitate a guy who'd been judged defective by at least three medical professionals, but he also had to hammer his way through a rock-hard wall of behavioral resistance. Like everyone else, there are things I like to do and things I say I'll do but probably won't. There was no point in giving me a training plan that I was going to half ignore, so Eric had to determine what kind of exercise I liked. He had no idea what he was in for.

"Do you belong to a gym?"

"Nope."

"What kind of workout equipment do you have at home?"

"None. I can't stand lifting. I can't stand anything that has to be counted or repeated. Waaay too monotonous."

I don't know why Eric didn't back out right then, but he soldiered on.

"Okay," he persevered. "What do you like?"

I paused for a sec, debating whether the truth would sound too weird or just plain useless. "You know those big old lumberjack saws?" I said. "The kind they used in the eighteen hundreds for taking down redwoods?"

"Yeah . . . ?"

"I have kind of an obsession with those. We heat our house with firewood, and a few years ago I stopped using the chain saw and started cutting all our wood with a crosscut. I should hate it—they call them 'misery whips'—but I could monkey around cutting wood all day. I've got, like, six saws."

"Okay," Eric replied. "We can work with that. . . ."

What Eric did next was simple brilliance—so brilliant, in fact, that it has taken me until now to figure it out. I was so excited by the trees—by Eric's training plan, his life-changing running technique, and his notion that runners have to be athletes first—that I missed the magnificence of the forest. Besides, like I said, there was that nude woman in there. I'm sure he tried to spell it out, but even if I'd listened, it was too radical a thought for me to have grasped at the time. Now that it's had a few years to sink in and I've also gotten used to the astounding change that Eric's approach has had on me, I'm finally able to appreciate what he's been trying to tell me, and what Jenni Blake discovered for herself out there in the Idaho wilderness.

And it's simply this: Humans love to move. Movement is in our genes; it's what has made us the most successful and widely traveled species on the planet (and beyond). To modern humans, though, that's a suspicious concept. We've been taught since birth to be suspicious of anything we enjoy, of anything that feels too much like fun, so we take what used to be joyful and playful and turn it into another form of work. No one says they're going to the gym to play, right? They're going to "work out."

But Eric knows that athleticism and achievement aren't about willpower. He's smart and honest enough to understand that anything you force yourself to do, at some point you'll stop doing. The self-discipline, no-pain-no-gain model just doesn't work, so instead, he's figured out a way to substitute pleasure for pain. He's helped bring a sense of artistry back to exercise, and for me, it's changed everything. Today, I'll walk out the door, look around, and pick a direction that seems appealing. Then I'll start to run, and I'll keep going as long and as far as I feel like—just the way I did when I was a kid. I won't worry about injuries, and I know my free time and water will give out before my energy. When I finish, I'll be eager to go again tomorrow.

And if you'd told me that five years ago, I'd have said it was impossible.

THE COOL IMPOSSIBLE

1

ME AND THE COOL IMPOSSIBLE

LET ME TELL you a story. . . .

In March 2006, I stood at the starting line of a fifty-mile race, living my Cool Impossible. Save for my dry-wick shirt and shorts, my hydration backpack, and the energy bars in my pockets, this was no ordinary race. Far, far from it. First, I was in the tiny remote village of Urique, tucked between steep cliffs and a river, in the Copper Canyon of northwestern Mexico. There was no grand race gate, no timer microchip on my shoes, no firing of a gun, and no massed swell of athletes tripping over one another to get ahead. There were only a couple dozen runners, a simple mark on the pavement in the center of town to indicate a starting point, and a tall, sun-bleached blond American nicknamed Caballo Blanco to shout, "Go!"

The runners that day were not my usual competitors either, and that was the point, really. This was a race to bring together two cultures, one old, one new, both with a devout love of running—and running at the extreme—over very long distances. In today's race, we faced fifty miles in the stark, hilly landscape of Copper Canyon.

Those of the new culture were among America's best ultramarathoners, including the dynamos Scott Jurek and Jenn Shelton. Two more experienced, iron-willed, and talented runners you'd be hard-pressed to find. They have the medals and championships to prove it.

Those of the older culture were the Tarahumara Indians. Dark and tawny skinned, their legs rippling with muscle, they wore loincloths and brightly colored long-sleeved shirts that billowed when they ran. Their shoes, or more appropriately huaraches, were simply a flattened, foot-shaped cutout of tire tread lashed to their feet with leather straps. The Tarahumara, whose true name is the Rarámuri (or "running people"), came from a collection of isolated, secret tribes who lived in Copper Canyon, surviving not much differently than they had for hundreds of years. They were known most of all for their amazing feats of endurance running, able to seemingly journey forever over parched and rocky trails across some of the most forbidding landscape on earth. I had known of their legendary feats for more than a decade, but to be with them in the flesh, as I had been for several days now, remained a wonder.

Then there were me and Christopher McDougall. Now, I had my share of ultraraces under my belt, but it was not like Scott eyed me with fear. Further, I had spent the months prior to the race changing diapers and rocking my new baby girl to sleep. My longest training run in advance of coming to Mexico clocked in at a paltry three hours, a third or less of the length of the run ahead of me that day. Finally, I was not just there as a competitor, but as a coach to Chris.

Alone among those at the starting line, Chris had never run an ultramarathon, and when we had first met a year before, he was a self-admitted "splintery wreck" who could not run a short distance without a long list of troubles. His original interest in the Tarahumara was as a journalist in the hunt for a good story. That had evolved since, and now he hoped to prove he could finish this very special ultramarathon race—for himself, for the idea of who he could be.

Beside me at the starting line, Chris was nervous and quiet and, typical of him, deflecting any attention paid by others to the rookie nature of his run. At six-foot-four, he's a big man, but was leaner by forty pounds since we began training together. "What'd you do to this guy?" Caballo had asked me on seeing the difference in Chris since their first meeting. Nonetheless, he was facing a fifty-mile run over treacherous, steep terrain in dry, scorching desert heat. I knew he could do it physically. The question was, Could he do it mentally? I'm sure he questioned both.

Moments before the race began, I told Chris, "Do your own thing; race your own race. Do what you know you can do, but if it feels like you're working, you're working too hard."

Soon after, Caballo shouted his "Go!" and we were off running. The Tarahumara exploded ahead at a blisteringly fast six-minute-mile pace, maybe faster. I was amazed and a bit flummoxed; could they possibly maintain that throughout the race? They were something to watch, smiles on their faces, their feet sprinting over the ground like they barely needed to touch it. They were out of earshot of the mariachi band, and out of Urique's town center, within seconds.

At a seven-minute pace, I followed, Chris still slower behind me. There was a long way to go, and as I told him, you have to run your own race. The first few miles were down a dirt road that stretched beside the Barranca River. I felt good, at ease for now, doing my own thing. We crossed a wood-and-rope suspension bridge, the whole contraption shaking and swinging as we traversed it single file. Soon after we started up our first big hill, a real leg burner, forty-five minutes in ascent, experiencing that special kind of excruciating joy that runners know better than most.

I could tell you that I came out of the womb shod with little baby running shoes, set to hit the trail. Or maybe that even in preschool I had a whistle around my neck, clipboard in hand, and was eager to coach. But both would be, well, fiction—and this story is true.

Like most of our journeys, mine zigzags, comes back on itself, and takes a few diversions. I actually arrived struggling for breath, my lungs attacked by asthma. My first Christmas was celebrated inside an oxygen tent. As a kid, I spent overnight birthday parties fighting for breath while my friends, full of cake and ice cream, slept easily. At an early age, I was very aware of my body, what it could do and not do. But my parents, my doctors, they never put barriers in front of me, forbidding this sport or that exercise. To this day I thank them, because the more I pushed myself, the more my body adapted and grew stronger.

In my small New York town in the hills of the Allegheny Mountains, I became a bit of a football star. Big fish, little pond. Classic. I was a running back who loved a crushing hit as much as a touchdown. Senior year of high school I ran track, chiefly to better my gridiron speed. To my surprise, I discovered the same joy I experienced on the football field, an awareness of my body's movement as an expression of who I was. Cue the chuckling, but I felt like an artist.

Two years of college football, graduation, and the cold-water splash of the real world came next. I had to build a life, put food on the table, find a home. The American West called, Denver specifically, and there at the edge of the Rockies, I ran, biked, swam, climbed, and kayaked in the fresh mountain air. I road-cycle raced, and competed in marathons, triathlons, adventure races, and ultraruns. I became a faster, stronger, better athlete than I ever imagined possible. But it was still a hobby. During the week, I clocked in at an environmental consulting firm. I was fine: interesting job, money in my pocket, a great view out my door, and adventure on the weekends. I had everything that I'd always wanted . . . and it wasn't what I *wanted*.

Through those years in Denver, above everything else, I lived and breathed running. And all without even really being sure where it was taking me. In time, though, I came to realize that I was never going to be *the best* runner. Still, I was a very good runner, and I had a lifetime's worth of athleticism woven deep into my bones. I started to think, How could I use the talents I was given—and that I had worked very hard to develop? I realized that I wanted to build my life around athletics—and that I wanted to help other people realize their own potential.

I quit my job, perks and all, and took a part-time one working the front desk at the University of Colorado Health Sciences Center fitness facility. I made a grand seven bucks an hour. Some people told me to "grow up," that I was following the wrong path. Forget them, I thought. I took classes in physiology, anatomy, biomechanics, and nutrition. I traveled to the U.S. Olympic Training Center in Colorado Springs and earned my credentials as one of the first USA Triathlon coaches. While still working at the fitness center, I began coaching one athlete, then another. Soon I had become the director of fitness at the UC center, and I collected a stable of runners and triathletes. Truth be told, I was learning as much as I was teaching.

Love and a commitment to help my wife, Michelle, care for her parents in Jackson, Wyoming, led to a decision to leave Denver. Don't anoint me with the title of saint, because selfishness and fear of losing the athletes I was coaching made the move a begrudged one. As would become clear, I better deserved the title of fool. In Jackson, in sight of the towering, jagged peaks of the Tetons, there was no better ultimate training environment, nor anyplace else so abounding with athletes literally hungry to be the fittest. I mean, there were world-class mountain-running trails right out my front door.

Amid this high-altitude, let's-go-attitude blend of enthusiasm and opportunity, my coaching career took off. I'd always told myself that it didn't matter if I had just one athlete; the important thing was to be living my life as a coach and runner. In Jackson Hole, I had an array of athletes in a wide range of events (plus I kept a bunch of my Colorado athletes, training them online), and the satisfaction was more than I'd ever imagined—just seeing my guys and girls improving week to week, sometimes session to session, was tremendously rewarding. And then there were the competitive successes, which in a lot of ways were even sweeter than the ones I'd experienced as an athlete myself. That list was growing: fifty- and hundred-mile-race champions in both running and mountain biking; age-group winners and podium finishers at run distances from 5K to 50K; Boston Marathon and Hawaii Ironman qualifiers; the silver medalist in the twenty-four-hour mountain-biking world championships; a Wyoming state high school cross-country champ; and even a professional hockey player, a few of Hollywood's fittest, and a rock-star guitar player. I was loving it—writing the workouts, designing the programs, figuring out the exercises—and other people were starting to notice, one in particular.

Like many tales, there's a proverbial knock on the door from a stranger in mine.

Or, more specifically, a phone call in 2005 from Chris McDougall. He wanted to do a feature on "America's best adventure workout," and I was, according to him, "the go-to conditioning guru in what is probably the most adventure sports–happy town in America." He had the second part right, at least. To save him from frostbite during the Wyoming winter, we met in Denver.

We hit it off, and I couldn't pry enough information out of him about the Tarahumara Indians, whom he had recently written about in *Runner's World.* A decade before, when one of their tribe raced for the first time in the Leadville Trail 100, a torturous ultramarathon in the heart of the Rockies, the Indian beat out all comers. For a time, I wanted to be a Tarahumara—or at least run like one. The whole idea of this tribe and their little-known world was part of what really got me into endurance. I was just drawn to it. It was so . . . primitive. And pure. I wanted to learn how that felt, that whole macrocycle of running these great distances and dealing with what goes on in your mind when you're out there running for five, eight, ten-plus hours. I loved the idea that I could go out and run all day like those Indians.

Now here was Chris, who had actually met them in the canyon lands and was thinking of running with them, at least for part of a fifty-mile race. Caballo Blanco, a mysterious and eccentric ultrarunner who had gone to live and run with the Tarahumara, was putting the event together.

But Chris was not in Denver to talk about the Tarahumara. He was there for an adventure workout, to learn how to build a body for multisport (kayaking, climbing, mountaineering) for an article.

To start, I took him out on a run in some low hills. He was an athletic guy, rowed in college, but he was very down about his ability to run. Basically, he said it was something he couldn't do because he suffered too much pain and didn't have enough endurance. He didn't like to train. In sum, he had given up.

That night I returned to the hotel, ripped apart our workout program, and decided to coach him as a runner. I knew anybody—big, small, fat, skinny, athletic or not—could transform him- or herself into an efficient runner. We met the next morning and I offered to help. I told him there was a right and a wrong way to run. He overstrode, suffered from a slow cadence, moved inefficiently, and struck the ground with his heels. Every step he took was breaking him down.

Throughout the next day, I introduced him to a new way to run and charted out a course for him to realize his overarching ambition: to run as many miles as he wanted on any given day for the rest of his life. At the end of our session, we sat on the green of the Denver City Park Golf Course and spoke about the Copper Canyon race. Chris said it was something he could never do, much as he wanted to run it. We made a gentlemen's bet: I would train him, and if he'd listen and do the work, I guaranteed him he could do the race. He then asked whether I'd join him in the run. "Yes" never came so quickly from my lips—well, except at my wedding.

Flash ahead a year, past some race-date hiccups, a newborn baby back home, and there I was in the state of Chihuahua, Mexico, jostling back and forth next to Chris in a rickety bus. We were descending six thousand feet to the town of Batopilas on a steep, one-lane dirt road pocked with holes. There was a cliff on one side, a rock wall on the other, and I feared we—this "dream team," as Caballo called us—would tumble to our deaths before meeting any of the running people.

Batopilas was the stepping-off point for our adventure. After two nights in a dingy hotel, we set off on a thirty-mile run/hike into the slotted canyons to reach the town of Urique, where the race was being held. We loaded our gear on mules, freeing ourselves to travel with only what we needed to drink and eat. Forty-five minutes into the journey, we came to a clearing shaded by a canopy of trees. Suddenly, we found ourselves surrounded by Tarahumara Indians. It was like they were ghosts, just materializing silently from the trees. Caballo introduced us by the spirit-animal names he had given us. I became El Gavilan, the hawk—quiet, confident, and ever watchful. Chris was Oso, the bear.

At once there was a very powerful sense of connection, a definite bond with the Tarahumara. We shared no language—we didn't know theirs; they didn't know ours. On that thirty-mile trek to the town of Urique, there was no talking. There were just expressions and gestures, but you could feel a kinship growing through our running. As we continued the journey, I closely observed the Tarahumara: their shoes, their running form, their strength, their bursts of speed, how they navigated the big rocks along the trail, and what they ate. They were amazing to watch, and I had to remind myself to keep my slack jaw from dragging across the dirt.

At last, we arrived in Urique after dark. In the few days before the race, we walked and ran some of the course, Caballo smirking whenever I asked him how hard he thought it would be. We ran more with the Tarahumara, had our own huaraches made from truck tires, demolished plates of fresh tortillas and tamales, and relaxed with beers at night. Truth be told, the scene was not much different from the simple mountain life centered around running that I had built for myself in Jackson.

After a restless night of sleep, race day came. In the morning, Chris, who always had a stash of espresso, shared a much-needed cup with me. I donned my jersey (number sixteen) and slipped on my hydration pack. The starting line awaited. Standing next to Chris, I knew he did not feel as though he deserved to be among this tribe, new and old, of endurance runners. The race would prove that for him, one way or the other.

Up canyons, through rivers, over hills, around turnabouts, down endless switchbacks, all through the heat and dust, mile after mile,

I ran. And I was hurting. The youngest of the Tarahumara, who had burst ahead at the start, were now slowing. Still, there was no way for me to PR (personal record) on this day, not the way I was feeling. I knew from the outset that I couldn't win this race, but I'm competitive, and I always want to feel like I am in the thick of the battle.

By mile eighteen—along a flat stretch of the trail, no less—I needed to stop. Something was off. My head wasn't in the race, and when you lose focus, it's easy to give in to the strain in the legs and lungs. By the trailside, I panted for breath, sweat pouring off me. Just then, Scott and the Tarahumara champion runner Arnulfo, who were coming around from a double-back, swept past me. Their sleek, supple legs were unfaltering, and so fast.

Right then I knew I needed to let go of this race as a competition and simply enjoy the run. The whole journey to Copper Canyon was part of a life centered around running that I had imagined for myself and worked to build for years, never allowing doubts or fears to stand in the way. That was the very essence of living the Cool Impossible, and winning this race had nothing to do with mine.

Coaching Chris, seeing him through the end of the Copper Canyon run, did. This experience in Mexico would remain unfulfilled, incomplete, unless he crossed the finish line—and crossed it running. Joining the tribe of endurance runners was his Cool Impossible, and I wanted it for him as part of my own.

At last, my focus in the right place, I returned to the trail feeling in the flow. I came down the long, steep hill that we had first climbed at the beginning. Feeling stronger and faster than I had earlier in the race, I was only a few miles from the finish.

Then, near the wood-and-rope suspension bridge, I came upon Chris. In last place, he was on his way toward the hill, at least two hours of running ahead of him. He was upbeat, but obviously feeling the effects of the heat and the miles. "The climb is going to seem a lot longer than you remember it. Be prepared," I told him, happy to see him still running. "These miles may seem like the longest in your life. Just settle in and run them."

Chris nodded and continued ahead. Throughout our training, I was never sure whether everything I said got through to him, but he was on his own now. Anything I could say, do, was already said and done.

After crossing the finish line in Urique—the same one that marked the start—I settled around a table at the town's lone restaurant with the other runners, Tarahumara and American alike. We drank, ate, and reveled in the race, rehashing it as runners always do. Then we ate, drank, and reveled some more. All the while, I thought of Chris, hoped he continued to place foot after foot across the trail.

Two hours later, twelve-plus hours since the race began, the sun was falling, the sky a brilliant orange, when word arrived that Chris was approaching. All of us, and our supporting mariachi band, gathered at the finish. I stared ahead, hoping to catch a first glimpse of him. Finally, Chris came down the road into the town square. He was running strong, enlivened by that last burst of adrenaline typical of the end of a race, even a really long one. I cheered. We all cheered, raising our fists, shouting, "Go, Oso! Go!"

Chris ran those fifty miles of brutal terrain. He ran them and joined the tribe of endurance runners. Once he crossed the finish line, he came up to me. Later he would tell me how much I helped him with that last bit of advice before he climbed that final big hill, but right now, at the finish, he was out of breath, too choked with thirst for words. We attempted a high five but missed. My excitement, his weariness—what can I tell you?—our aim was off. But then he grabbed my hand in that big paw of his own and squeezed it tight. I could feel the joy in the embrace, and there was nothing left to say.

With my coaching, Chris achieved his own Cool Impossible. I'm proud to say many of my athletes have done the same, and I'm here, fired up and ready, to guide you to your own.

2

YOU IN GLORIOUS JACKSON HOLE

OKAY. ENOUGH ABOUT me and the near past.

This is about you and your near future. You, the athlete—and I use that word with full consideration and intent. Because wherever you are in your running life, you can make the choice to be an athlete. You can adopt that mind-set and make it your own defining essence. Being an athlete *is not* something you're "born with." That's a misconception, a myth, really, that is all too often also an impediment—or, even worse, an excuse. Being an athlete *is* a choice. And making that choice, taking up that mind-set, is the step that allows you to move toward a new level of achievement. That's what this book is about. And that's what I'm going to ask of you.

The truth is, athleticism is awareness. That simple phrase is at the core of my program. When I say, "Athleticism is awareness," what I mean is that to be an athlete means you are someone who is aware of your form and technique; aware of how you move your body; aware of your effort level, of your breathing pattern; aware of what you eat (and don't eat); and, most important, aware of what you think (and don't think).

We will go deeper into that idea later, but first we need to address the physical side of things. I believe firmly that the mind follows the body. And when the mind follows a good body, it gets to the right place. So that is where we will begin the journey—your journey—to the Cool Impossible.

To get started, I am going to ask you to look at things maybe a little differently than you've looked at them in the past. I'm going to introduce you to some new ideas and concepts and ask you to do some new things that will help to catapult your running to another level and help you get everything that you want out of every mile. Along the way, I am going to challenge you to go above and beyond what you think is possible for yourself, for your running, and, I hope, even your life.

And to be clear, this process, this challenge—this opportunity—is open to every runner. This book is for you whether you're a beginner, or a veteran hoping to reclaim that beginner's enthusiasm and sense of possibility; whether you're a dedicated competitor, gearing your efforts to improvements in time and placings at key races, or a recreational runner, excited about the social aspects of the sport; whether you're someone whose running has been interrupted or compromised by chronic injury, or an enthusiastic experimenter inspired by visions of barefoot running, the Tarahumara Indians, and other adventures. This commitment to awareness will—like Frost's choice between two roads diverging in a wood—make all the difference.

One element of what you will learn later is how important and powerful a role visualization plays in performance. The mind follows the body and, in turn, performance follows the mind. But harnessing that sequence, controlling it and making it work for us to carry us to where we want to go, is a challenge—and one that often goes unrecognized. We have lost touch with the art of daydreaming. I don't mean the kind of daydreaming that comes after a few hours of surfing vacation Web sites or buying that lottery ticket. We're all pretty good at that. No, I mean the kind of daydreaming that can help guide our performance and prepare us for the journey to the Cool Impossible.

So let's give it a try. Let's do it. Right now. Rather than simply telling you what's going to come in the chapters ahead—laying out the programs and the protocols, explaining the mechanics, the physiology and the psychology—I'm going to give you a chance to live it. I wake up each day in Jackson thrilled anew to find myself in what is truly a running and adventure-sport paradise, living the kind of life that I once could only imagine. But that's the point: I *did* imagine it, and now it's as real as the vast, jagged face of the Teton Range that beckons me each time I step out of my house, or the bear that ambles across the trail ahead of me on my morning run, or the lung-searing challenge of an uphill sprint at nine thousand feet. I want to make it just as real for you.

I want you to imagine that you are on your way to visit me in Jackson Hole for an intense seven-day running camp. This one-on-one camp will be like no other running you've ever done and will introduce you to and immerse you in every element of my training program. Jackson Hole is the real deal, the true Wild West. It's here that you can find your own frontier and be shocked into a new reality. I am hoping this is what you expect from your visit and from this book, because it is what I want for you.

So, here you are. . . . It's been a short flight from Denver or Salt Lake City (or wherever you made your connection, because, face it, unless you've got a private jet you're not flying direct to Jackson). But it is a leap into another realm. The plane drops down out of the clouds and suddenly there it all is, a landscape so sweeping and majestic that it makes you almost laugh as you press your face to the little square of the window: the mountains, saw edged and brilliantly snowcapped, marching out to the horizon; the Snake River running its sinuous course through the valleys; the burnished tans and greens of the headlands. We are most certainly not in Kansas (in real or metaphorical terms) anymore.

You can see immediately why they call it Jackson *Hole*. The floor of the valley sits at sixty-five hundred feet, but the Tetons on the western side soar like a wall to thirteen thousand feet, and the Gros Ventre Range to the east tops out near twelve thousand feet. Trappers and hunters who found their way to the region in the early nineteenth century must have felt they were literally going over the edge as they climbed down the steep canyons into the vast encircled expanse. It still feels that way today, as the plane drops down, far below the peaks, and settles in for a landing at Jackson Hole Airport, which, with its low-slung rustic design, seems to blend in with the flat expanse of the valley.

No Jetway here. You grab your bag, running shoes dangling from the handle, and exit the plane directly onto the tarmac. You take a deep breath. The air is exhilarating and the sky astoundingly wide and close. As you follow the concrete path toward the terminal, you turn to look at the mountains, and it's like they're right there in your face. Your eye traces the wild, zigzag lines of the peaks—dominated by the central massif, the truly majestic Grand Teton—and follows the canyons cutting up in deep, dark Vs between the rises. You try to imagine running there, following a trail up to the Teton Crest. It seems like another world. Another you, perhaps.

Welcome to Jackson: That sort of spectacular vista, with its promise and its challenge, is everywhere here. It is also the reason why *you're* here. In the next few days you're going to get a firsthand taste of all that Jackson has to offer, and at the same time an introduction to my running program, a taste of what I'll be asking you to do, and a glimpse of where these new elements and new ways of thinking can take you—in your running and in your life.

We meet outside the airport. I'm the shaved-headed, skinny guy with rounded shoulders and a cheery smile. I'm happy to see you, after all. I bundle you into my truck and off we go, windows down.

On the ride into town from the airport we pass buffalo—yep, they're roaming—beside the road, as well as an elk framed against the sky above a ridge, the same ridge on which we'll put in some quality miles in the days to come. We also pass a trio of cyclists, pulling big gears as they roll down the shoulder not that much slower than we're driving. You'll learn that it's impossible to go for long in Jackson Hole without seeing someone in motion: biking, running, hiking, paddling on the streams, skiing the trails in winter. The most adventure sports–happy town in America—Chris had it right.

But on this first night, before we move into action, there's time to sit and talk, to get a sense of where you're coming from, and where *we're* going to be going in the course of the next seven days—and beyond. Over a steak salad or grilled trout at the Snake River Brewery, we'll talk about a lot of things. About Jackson, and the history of the valley. About the Wild West. About skiing at lunchtime and about what twenty-below really feels like. About crazy real-estate prices and about mountain lions. Behind it all, of course, will be that sense of anticipation, of an adventure about to be embarked upon. Maybe you're a little tired or fried from the travel, but you're feeling a buzz, too, that tingle that every runner knows that precedes a big test. And so we'll start talking about the aspects of your upcoming training. Since I'm a bottom-up kind of guy, we'll start with your feet.

Don't worry, we're not going all Barefoot Ted here. My Copper Canyon race companion, and one of the pioneers of barefoot running, has a lot of wisdom to share, but I consider shoeless running a tool—something that can help build strength and improve form for all runners—rather than as an objective in and of itself, or even, as some would have it, a lifestyle. Remember, the Tarahumara sport those huaraches, not bare feet, across their rocky trails. For now, we're going to concentrate on strengthening the feet, and it's crucial that you can feel—really *feel*—what we're doing.

Take your shoes off. It's okay—we're in Jackson here; you won't be the first at this establishment. Now look down at those feet, maybe a little pale below the sock line, the toes spreading and gripping the tile floor. For all the usual focus on leg strength, flexibility, and core fitness, when it comes to running, everything springs, quite literally, from those two kind of funny-looking appendages. Just as a race car, no matter how big an engine it has or how sophisticated a suspension, depends on four small patches of tire on asphalt to get around a track, a runner's performance and health are rooted in the actions of the foot, with its twenty-six bones, thirty-three joints, and more than a hundred muscles, tendons, and ligaments. Having strong feet promotes proper muscle usage all the way up the leg and throughout the core, ultimately creating the muscle equilibrium that is so important to successful running, and that's what we'll be working on throughout your training.

Maybe you're imagining a gym full of machines and clanking iron; maybe you sneaked a peek down at your biceps last time you raised your glass, or you're trying to remember how much you hoisted the last time you did heavy leg squats. But strength training is not about how much you can lift. That's not the challenge. The challenge is to have an open mind about what the objective is. Strength training is about muscle equilibrium—about making sure that the big, prime-mover muscles in the body don't overwhelm the smaller supporting muscles, pulling the entire system out of balance and compromising efficiency. It's more important how well we move and how efficient we are in using our strength than how much weight we can toss around.

And the amazing thing is that this muscle equilibrium, this *athletic* strength, will help you to run better. It will also prevent the all too familiar aches and pains and stiffness that can sometimes seem like the unavoidable price of running.

Let me be very clear about this: These aches, these pains, they are avoidable. You may have been conditioned to think otherwise, but over the course of our time together, I will show you different. With strength, muscle equilibrium, good form, and a proper training program, we can eliminate those common running ailments, have more fun, and achieve tremendous performance enhancements.

Easy, now; I don't want to overwhelm you. Let's pay the check, take a walk down Town Square. It's not Times Square, New York City, but what we lack in glittering lights, we make up for in quiet charm and a backdrop that takes the breath away.

I want to know some more about you. If you're shy, don't be. This is important. Before I begin coaching any athlete, I like to get a detailed sense of where he is in his running career. We runners love to talk running. It's our currency of exchange, as natural as putting one foot in front of the other. So let's talk about past races, the good ones and the ones that kicked our butts. Let's talk about workouts and recent long runs; tell me about your favorite route and how fast you've covered it recently. And in the process I'll get a sense of your experience level and where you are in your training. And I'll ask you—just as you no doubt are asking yourself—what your goals are. What do you want out of your running—from the season ahead, in terms of a specific race or training goal, to a lifetime ahead on the road or trails? If you are not a racer, we can discuss how races can personally empower you and foster a sense of adventure in your running.

Okay, that's a lot of talk and very little action. It'd be nice to grab a beer together—or, if that's not your thing, a coffee or tea. But this first night, it shouldn't be a late one. We've got a whole week ahead of us, and it's time to turn in. I'll file away what I've gleaned about your running past and your goals for the future.

Back at your hotel, you settle in to sleep, your window open to the cool mountain air and all that awaits outside on the trails of Jackson.

An hour after sunrise, the steep slopes of the Tetons are sharply etched in soaring lines of light and shadow, and the rolling foothills are rising into burnished greens and gold. We meet at the Cache Creek Canyon trailhead. A popular hiking, biking, and cross-country trail that runs along Cache Creek close to downtown Jackson, this will be an ideal setting for a short shakeout run. This is not a workout. It's just to get the blood flowing, an easy, roly-poly outing in the woods, a chance for you to get acclimated to the altitude and for me to watch you run.

We'll go for thirty-five to forty minutes, whatever feels comfortable. I'll keep the instructions intentionally vague at the beginning—nothing more complicated or nuanced than, "Take it easy"—since the important thing is to get a sense of how you naturally run. I'll be watching your form, and to do that I'll move around on the trail, leading for a while and then dropping back to follow. I might speed up the pace for a stretch and then slow it back down. I'll be looking to see how you respond: Do you push to keep up—despite those instructions at the start to keep it easy? Or do you do your own thing? I'll be looking to see how confident you are in your own pace.

You can learn a vast amount about people just by going on an easy run with them. Every step reveals a wealth of detail, and I'm making notes in my head as we go along: *Hey, her pace is good*, or *Hmm, his stride crosses over*; *He's not using his glutes*; or *She's a heel striker*. All of this gives me a road map for going forward.

I'm an expert at running and talking—comes with the job. So let me cover a little about form as we go. Like I told Chris, there's a right and a wrong way to run, and I'm here to teach you the difference. The specifics will come later. For now, let's address the significance of form.

When we have good form, we run efficiently. With bad form . . . wait for it . . . you're running inefficiently. Bad form forces you to use some muscles more, and others less, than is optimal. Over time, the ones we use strengthen; the ones we don't weaken. It's not rocket science. This disparity throws off the body equilibrium I told you about before. When that happens, you create tightness in your muscles, and you suffer from common running ailments in your hips, knees, ankles, and feet. We'll focus a lot on form, and I'm confident that once you start making changes, you'll like the transformation in your running.

But right now, it's important that we make sure the run stays relaxed and natural, to keep you from becoming self-conscious. The hardest thing for a person to do is to run as he or she normally does when she knows there's someone watching. Of course, there's a good chance you'll be a bit distracted—by the scenery of Jackson, with the woods just waking to the day, the mountains coming into focus beyond the trees; by the thoughts of what you're going to be asked to do over the next seven days; and, of course, by the altitude.

If you're coming from sea level, this first run at six thousand feet is going to be a real eye-opener, and not just in the good-morning sense. You'll feel it just walking from the car to the trailhead: that sense that each breath is bringing in just a tiny bit less oxygen than you need. Even at a relaxed pace on the trails, a sense of desperation can creep in, as each slight rise brings a gasping moment of oxygen debt. Yeah, yeah, Jackson is gorgeous, and the morning sun through the trees is amazing, and we might see a bear or a mountain lion or who knows what else, but right about ten minutes into this easy run, your vision is narrowed to the single track in front of you, and your thoughts are on nothing more than the next step. This is a shakeout run? It feels more like a survival test. But you press on. That's what you're here for. And the amazing thing is how the body always adapts. Even by the end of this first short outing, you'll feel a bit stronger, like there's more you can give. And that, right there, is part of the process.

As we slow to a jog and then a walk on the last switchbacks down to the trailhead, your pulse rate and breathing returning to normal, you're already thinking ahead to the next run, considering how you'll respond to a greater challenge. You're eager, excited, energized.

This is a good time for me to hit you with the heart and soul of my program. Sometimes I call it cardiovascular training, because there's a lot of pumping blood and heaving lungs during its execution. But there's much more that happens during this aspect of your training—improving running efficiency, developing strength, burning fat, raising lactic acid thresholds, getting faster—and so you'll also hear me address it as your "strategic running foundation." Catchphrase or not, what I'll lay out for you with a specific day-by-day schedule is a system of training runs focused on either speed or heart-rate zones.

Following it will build for you a foundation of endurance, speed, and strength for whatever kind of running you want to do, no matter what level of runner you are. This program is flexible and dynamic enough to work for the beginner simply looking to develop a healthy approach to running, to the experienced competitor who's hitting a plateau, and to those who are looking to run their first 5K, 10K, half marathon, marathon, or beyond.

Gets you hungry just thinking about it, right?

Next stop is breakfast. We'll roll back into town and hit the Bunnery, just off Town Square, bright and bustling with folks off to work and others in from their morning workouts—rides and runs and climbs and paddles. There's nothing like sitting down to breakfast knowing that you've already done a morning run. The engine is fired and ready for fuel.

This will be a good time to talk a bit about nutrition—surrounded by the aroma of fresh-baked muffins and buns, breakfast burritos, and blueberry pancakes. Nutrition is a very important part of my program (something you'll learn over the next few days), though not so much in terms of day-by-day, meal-by-meal schedules and menus. It's not about becoming a label (vegan, paleo, veggie). To me, the question of nutrition is more about mind-set: With the commitment to becoming an athlete, and living as an athlete, comes the sense that you live with awareness. That includes awareness of what you put in your mouth. We will talk about natural eating, and avoiding processed foods, and particularly sugar. But mainly the message is that we all *know* what we should be eating, and, just as important, what we shouldn't be eating. The key is to stop taking half measures and just do it right. Oh, and pass the salsa for the huevos rancheros.

Breakfast is over—a lot to digest so far in many ways. Go rest, take a siesta at your hotel, maybe head out for a leisurely walk afterward. Take in a bit of Jackson, talk to some locals, get a feel for the place where you'll be spending the next week. I'll pick you up when the sun is on its wane.

It's late afternoon, and we're back in the truck, bombing north past the airport into Grand Teton National Park. We turn in at Moose Junction and cross the Snake River, shadows from the falling sun now stretching across its waters. We follow Teton Park Road farther up into the park. There's still a nice warmth in the air, but you can't help but notice the narrow poles flashing past at regular intervals along the side of the road. They're there to mark the edge of the pavement when the route is covered in snow—and they're taller than the truck. What, you wonder, looking out through the greens and browns of the woods, must it be like here in the winter, when all is white?

While your mind is wandering to thoughts of taking up ski mountaineering, or snow biking, we pull in and park beside the eastern edge of Jenny Lake.

This is where we're going to do another run, and it is a spot unlike any you've ever seen. Formed by glaciers twelve thousand years ago and framed by the tallest peaks in the Teton Range, Jenny Lake is about two miles long and a mile wide at the middle, and its crystal water mirrors the sky and the mountains perfectly. For the next hour or so, this living postcard will form the backdrop to our workout, even as you're going to be focusing not outward on the scenery, but inward on your own mental landscape.

As we take off along the pine-needle trail around the lake, I want you to think about the importance of training the mind, as well as the body. Thinking affects performance, period. I'll talk a lot about this over the coming days, but for now, I just want to further introduce this idea of awareness.

With awareness comes the possibility of control and improvement, of progress and mastery—and, ultimately, of new possibility. In many ways, actually, *what* we think is not what's important. What *is* important is our awareness of our thinking, and, then, how we act after we think it. It's human nature, for instance, to want to know what's in store, to ask before we attempt something, "What's going to happen? What is the outcome going to be?" Our thinking—this need to "know"—is often what stops us from doing the things we want to do, or dream of doing, especially when we're not sure we can. Call it a fear of the unknown. It can stop us before we start. But if we can identify that fear—if we have *awareness* of it—and still go forward, then we're on a clear road to our dreams. Crazy things happen when you're on that road. Crazy good things. That's something that I've learned over the course of my life, and it has become the foundation for my own athletic endeavors and for my philosophy of training. When we embark on any venture—whether it's running or any other endeavor in life—it's crucial that we don't get hung up about the outcome. Yes, every athlete has his or her goals, and it's important and necessary to aim for those. But we don't know how it's going to turn out, and that's the glory.

This is not all loose theory (i.e., "Here's what's theoretically possible, but you're on your own to figure out how to obtain it"). No. There are specific techniques you'll learn from me. The journey begins by helping you identify your goals, what it is you actually want to accomplish as a runner. You've done some visualization already with me, but there's much more to come.

I'll also teach you how to use mantras. Don't worry: I'm not talking sitting like Buddha, legs crossed, incense swirling around your head, and humming deeply "om" after "om." That's great, if that's your thing. But mantras come in all different shapes and sizes. They can simply be repeating phrase like, "Do what's required." Their power comes in focusing your thoughts, centering your mind to your purpose.

Heady stuff, quite literally, but if you trust me to lead you through every step of the Cool Impossible, you'll see that it works.

Now slow down; come and sit beside me on the lakeshore. Good. Now, I know what you're thinking: Go ahead—take your shoes off; I know you want to slip those tired feet into the cold blue water of Jenny Lake. Nice, right? Hopefully, you feel a kind of open flow through your body, a relaxed sense of connectedness.

We sit here awhile, not speaking, just taking it all in.

There—look up now into the wide blue Wyoming sky. There, far, far above, a bald eagle is circling, riding the currents seemingly effortlessly, everything—anything—within its reach. Maybe, you think, you can relate.

3

TRUE STRENGTH

OKAY, TIME TO turn to the training, starting with strength. You've settled into Jackson Hole. Maybe you've not yet acclimated to the altitude, but hopefully you feel eager and ready to go deeper into reaching your own Cool Impossible.

We meet at Snow King Resort, a short run from Town Square. This is where the locals come to ski. The paint on the lift towers may be chipped, but who cares? We're talking fifteen hundred feet of vertical in less than two miles. Steep. Outside of winter, the resort is a different kind of adventure center. Today, mountain bikers hitch a lift up the mountain for the ride of their lives down. Hikers follow the trails into the dense pine forests. Paragliders swoop through the sky. And, not far from where we settle in to talk at a picnic table, a trio of climbers hit the bouldering park. Look at them using their bodies: so much awareness, so much useful strength. We can learn a lot from climbers. You will.

For a moment, let's step back from our visualization. If you were really to come out to Jackson and join me for a one-on-one session, I'd teach you about strength, form, strategic running foundation, nutrition, awareness, and training the mind all together. But we have time in this book, so why rush? Each chapter, we'll zero in on one element in depth. I'll give you the theory, the why and how we focus on each aspect, then provide a specific program to follow. Remember, though, these lessons are not separate and distinct from one another. Strength helps form, form helps strength, and you could say the same for every element. One last note—or suggestion. Before executing any of the specific programs (for instance, the foot strength exercises to come in this chapter), please read through the whole book; then back up again and dive into each.

The structure of the book is meant to work best if you have an overview of the whole plan first. Then, optimally, you will begin the strength exercises while working on form (and the transition/rejuvenation program), followed by the strategic running foundation program. Nutrition and awareness you can implement and practice throughout.

Finally, later in the book, I'll teach you how to self-coach and to listen to your body to remain feeling good and train within your ability. It's also important to note that you should start this training program only when you're feeling good and are injury-free. If you have questions or uncertainty about your health, please consult with a doctor and/or physical therapist before launching into my program.

Okay, you're at Snow King again. Six days left to go in Jackson, and we're first focusing on strength. Strange, you might say, strength first? How can we do strength training at a park at the base of a ski hill? And don't I, like many runners, get enough "nonrunning" training with cross-fit exercises or the like?

Lots of questions. Good, that shows you're interested.

First, trust me. Second, remember strength helps form and vice versa. Third, understand that my strength program develops your overall athleticism. Finally—and I've saved the best for last—long hours in the gym aren't the way to achieve athleticism. I know you like to run, and the potent strength exercises I recommend will allow you to have plenty of time to devote to hitting the trail.

So, over the day, I'll explain exactly what I mean by strength, how/

where we need to build it throughout the body, and the role of awareness in that process, and finally we'll run through a regimen of exercises. At the end of this session, you'll know your body—and feel it—in profoundly new ways.

A NEW IDEA OF STRENGTH

Throw away your preconceived notions of strength. We are not talking about heavy lifting, drifting between exercises at the gym, or fighting for space in Monday morning's sculpt or cross-fit class. These all serve a purpose for a variety of personal reasons, but I challenge you to think differently about what a strong body should be for you as a runner. Remember, the Tarahumara Indians are not only great runners, but they're also great athletes.

For me, strength is the ability to use stored-up energy in our muscles, to create power, to propel and stabilize movement as efficiently as possible. It is the ability to use energy to accomplish a task through time. As runners, we want to cover a distance, often a long one, with enduring speed. We don't want to fatigue, and we don't want to break down and lose form. All that requires strength.

Integral to this idea of strength is equilibrium. We want the whole body to act and perform as a single unit, and we develop efficiency by using the body "well" and training it to be balanced. Developing muscle equilibrium eliminates what I call big-muscle dominance (think of your quads or chest) by fostering those small, supporting muscles (think of the muscles in your ankles, hips, and spine) that often go underutilized. Equilibrium promotes movement, stability, endurance, and power.

In my experience as a coach, I have too often seen runners, those who work on strength at all, focus on building these bigger, prime mover muscles. This only accentuates their dominance, pushes others to grow weak or dormant, and furthers an imbalance in the body that might have already been developed over time from poor form and other issues. Disequilibrium causes tightness and leads to those all too familiar running troubles: tight hip flexors, hamstrings, IT band pain, Achilles trouble, low-back pain, poor breathing, runner's knees, stiff upper body, rounded shoulders, and poor biomechanics.

Speaking of tightness, let me say again: Chronically tight muscles come from muscle dominance and unequal muscle activation. If you have equilibrium, you should not be chronically tight. Therefore (and this may surprise you, because it goes against popular wisdom), we should not need to stretch excessively. Excessive tightness is telling you something, and stretching may help it feel better, but will not take care of the problem.

Remember, there's a certain part of tightness in muscles that is required to be fast and powerful, to have strength. The classic analogy is a rubber band. If you stretch a rubber band too far, it loses its elasticity and becomes useless. We want the rubber band taut and snappy. It's the same with how we want our muscles. They store energy and act as springs to release energy. That's power and speed. That's healthy.

Once and for all, we need to stop thinking of strength in terms of how much we can lift, how hard we can work, how quickly we can get through this circuit, or working so hard we lose form. Instead, we need to focus on equilibrium by activating dormant muscles, and creating neuromuscular pathways to help fire more muscles. Stop thinking that a strong core is an end in and of itself. Instead, think about how we activate our core during movement and running. The same can be said of our feet, calves, hamstrings, quads, and arms.

Athleticism is many things that come together at once. It's about moving well and efficiently. It is about controlling this movement through an awareness of what your body is doing in space and action, and how its individual parts are working together. Through strength training, you create stability and equilibrium among these individual parts, allowing them to work seamlessly, powerfully, with one another to achieve your goals as an athlete.

Now, you want to see athleticism, true strength. Take a look over there at the bouldering park; watch those climbers, their hands dusted with chalk, straining for the next hold. Notice their sinewy arms and legs. Watch how they use leverage, balancing from one side of their body to the other, always aware of where they are, where they're going. They're precise in their movements, yet still at ease, actively realizing that perfect balance of power and relaxation. Pound for pound, inch for inch, climbers can boast of being the strongest, most efficient, and most balanced athletes on the planet. They are pure, lean power incarnate, able to harness anaerobic capabilities with aerobic endurance. That's what we want to build for you from the ground up, and I mean that literally.

TRUE STRENGTH—FROM THE GROUND UP

Foot and Leg Strength

Let's stand up. Get away from the picnic table and take those shoes and socks off. As you do so, maybe you're wondering about the contraption I've just pulled out of my gym bag. That five-by-five-inch wood board with a single leg at the end that resembles a small ramp? That's a slant board. The round board, five inches in diameter, with a sawed-off ball of wood at its bottom is a stability disk. The ski poles, which you already gave me an odd look for bringing, are to help you balance on one foot on top of these boards. These are the tools you will use to develop foot/leg strength in the exercise program to follow.

Yes, your feet. It's rare for people to talk about runners needing to be athletic—and the strength that comes with that. It's rarer still for foot strength to be in the conversation. Bizarre, really, since the design of our feet, from toes, to arch, to heel, is integral to our ability to run. You could argue that they were essential to our ability to survive—and thrive—back in our days as hunter-gatherers. Our feet, with their many bones, joints and muscles, tendons, and ligaments, are key to athletic strength and equilibrium. Most athletes don't think—it's simply not in our consciousness—that we can train our feet, but we can, and we should think of doing so with the same level of purposefulness that we pay to "the core."

For runners, the feet are more than a key part of our strength. Everything starts with them. They set the stage, good or bad, for the whole leg, and we want to set a very, very good stage.

So why did I ask you to take your shoes off at the beginning? I'm not a zealot who feels that running barefoot is the answer to all your troubles. That said, I always train my athletes barefoot during strength training. Shoes can inhibit natural movement, and they definitely get in the way of your feeling the ground. As we work on you from the feet up, it's critical to be aware of how you use your feet and how they affect your ability to perform. Going shoeless is critical while executing the exercises.

Speaking of shoes: When you were last in a store to buy some, were you told that you had flat feet or overpronate (roll your feet to the inside with each stride) or supinate (roll to the outside)? If so, you're not the first. Often the clerk, well-intentioned though he may be, will say you need this kind of shoe or that kind of orthotic to compensate for your issue. He's wrong. Overpronation, supination, these are fundamentally about a lack of foot stability, and therefore, developing your foot strength will likely prove to be the only orthotic—and a natural one, to boot—that you'll need. Same with flat feet. I used to suffer from a very low arch. My regimen of foot strength exercises gave me a strong, high arch.

For the moment, forget the slant board and stability disk. Let's just do a quick test of your foot strength. Balance on one foot. Maybe it's challenging, but not too difficult? Now balance only on your forefoot, your heel off the ground. Try to maintain that position for thirty seconds. Not as easy as you thought, right? You probably had to fight for your balance without your arch collapsing—that's if you were able to keep the heels off the ground for much time at all.

Okay, come back and sit down. If you need to, rub those feet. I have more explaining to do.

A lack of foot strength reduces our stability, and stability is the foundation you need to propel yourself forward efficiently. Without it, you are no different from a house with a weak structure. Over time, things will collapse. That's to my point about how foot strength sets the stage for everything else. It does so because of its interconnectedness to the rest of your lower body, from your ankles, calves, and knees to your glutes. When you were balancing on your forefoot, did you feel a slow burn moving up your calves, perhaps in your butt? Case closed.

As runners, this interconnection makes it impossible to separate foot strength from leg strength. Utilizing the foot properly (due to strength, awareness, and good form) promotes what I call muscle activation up the leg and creates muscle equilibrium. By training the foot, you allow the muscles in the leg to fire as they should. This activates more muscle fibers, creating economy and efficiency. It is not about building bigger muscles; rather, it is about inviting more muscles and fibers to the party to create more strength, power, and stability.

To flash forward, when you first begin the program of exercises I'll show you soon with the slant board, you will likely find that your feet suffer the brunt of the strain. However, as you develop foot strength, this allows more muscles to fire in the calves and up to your glutes, and you'll start to feel a good burn there rather than in your feet. In other words, you'll get it where you need it.

Granted, I may already have you sold on the foot-leg-strength dynamic, but as further illustration, I want to give you a specific and too common issue that occurs when we don't have proper strength at the foundation. It is emblematic of the fact that all of our aches and injuries from running are not normal and simply don't have to exist. You'll see the truth of that as we continue throughout our time together.

The gluteus medius muscle is located on your hip (think that spot between the front and back pocket of your jeans). It's the big kahuna when it comes to running stability. Weakness—or, more specifically, poor activation of the gluteus medius—is the most frequent culprit I find inhibiting an athlete's optimal performance or causing pain. Yet again, the effectiveness of our gluteus medius begins with the feet.

In an ideal body with ideal form, the forefoot strikes the ground first in the running stride. The big toe and arch help stabilize the rest of the foot, and your heel comes down to the ground. Then you toe off with your forefoot, your heel elevates, and your calves fire. The ankle and knee remain in alignment, the quads and hamstrings do their jobs, and your gluteus medius activates to stabilize your hips as you propel forward. You run straight and strong.

Now, in a less ideal, more common world, our feet often lack proper strength. A parade of problems follows. Our heels don't elevate as they should, our ankles and knees come out of alignment, the calves don't fire well, our quads overwork, and the gluteus medius is not activated.

When the gluteus medius fails in its chief task to stabilize our body as we run, our hips go left and right. You may not see or feel that movement, but it's there for many runners. The hip flexors are called into action to aid in stabilization, a job for which they are not designed. Instead, they're meant to lift the leg. But when called to duty otherwise, they will pitch in to stabilize, to their own detriment (and yours).

Over time in this less than ideal world, we further destabilize as some muscles (namely the quads and hip flexors) become dominant and tight from overuse. Meanwhile, the calves and gluteus medius weaken from disuse. Watch out then. Here comes hip pain, shin splints, runner's knees, and Achilles trouble.

Do you have IT band pain, or have you been told all your issues come from the same? Well, this tightness often comes from using our quads too much. When the quads overwork, this creates stress on the fibers of the IT band and the quad muscles that attach to the knee. Boom—knee pain.

Seldom do you find the area of pain, discomfort, or tightness to be the same as its source. Yet over and over, we treat the area, not the source. We don't have to be broken-down runners and tight all the time. Work on strength, first with the feet, and break the cycle that breaks us down.

I may have spent a lot of time talking about pain or injuries. And yes, many of you, I'm sure, have these troubling issues. But I'm also sure there are an equal number of you who aren't injured, don't have pain. That's great. But don't lose sight of the importance of developing proper foot and leg strength. Doing so will create more economy and efficiency in your running. It will improve performance. Period.

So, all of you, create a new cycle, one that promotes muscle equilibrium and stability, and you will run faster, more efficiently, and with less pain or tightness, gathering more strength as you go. Rock on, I say.

Paragons of Strength—The Tarahumara Indians

While in Urique the days before the Copper Canyon race, I spent every possible moment watching and interacting with the Tarahumara. I wanted to know how they'd become such amazing endurance runners. What gave them the ability to run a hundred miles, more, in a single day over such extreme terrain?

I found their special "sauce." It's not some extra muscle or anatomical advantage. It's many ingredients blended together: running early and a lot as children, their diet, their terrain, their shoes, the games they play running, a whole lifestyle built around movement. But this sauce isn't magical or surprising. Much of what I observed in the Tarahumara I had already come to learn was essential for my own athletes. Rather than being revelatory, my time in Mexico was more affirming of the new "sauce" I had developed in my own coaching. That said, in the field of coaching runners, one that is both an art and a science, affirmation is a beautiful, powerful thing.

In terms of strength, the Tarahumara have it in all the right ways for endurance running. This first became clear

(cont.)

to me when Manuel, who is a kind of grandfather of the tribe of Indians, offered to make Barefoot Ted his own pair of huaraches. In his late fifties, sporting a Yankees baseball cap over his still jet-black hair, Manuel had run in the first Leadville race featuring the Tarahumara.

While making Ted's pair of huaraches, he remained in a squat on the side of the main street in Urique. Feet square, his butt sitting low, almost touching the ground, he sawed away at the old tire tread with his serrated knife. Not a big deal, you say. Attempt a simple deep squat on your own; see how close you can bring your butt to the floor in a squat without your knees going inward. Or maybe your squat is more like a lean at the waist. Manuel's ability to remain in a squat for close to an hour while working with his hands demonstrated remarkable stability, mobility, and muscle equilibrium.

In the following days, as we ran the same trails that Manuel and the other Tarahumara ran, there was no doubt where he had developed this strength—and it reinforces my belief in the central role that our feet play in athleticism. The trails through the steep canyons around Urique are far from the well-tended, frequently traveled paths that we are accustomed to in the United States. They're rough, uneven, and strewn with rocks and boulders of every size and shape. To run along these trails demands not only your attention, but also the ability for your feet to land on rocks at various angles, and then toe off to advance forward.

Further, when crossing the Copper Canyon terrain, it's rare for both feet to be landing on level terrain. More often, I found myself landing with one foot on a slanted rock, then another on the path. This requires balance, lunging, and squatting. The Tarahumara do this kind of running repeatedly, day after day, on long runs, up and down mountains. They do so in their worn-out flat huaraches, their feet and calves the only shock absorbers they have. In extremely rocky stretches, they're basically doing one-legged squats while running fast. They've trained their bodies to move strong and powerfully with incredible stability, and it comes naturally. No heavy weights, no slow lifting techniques concentrating on a single muscle.

In many ways, my program of exercises on the slant board and stability disk re-creates the movements and demands on the feet and legs that I saw Manuel and others experience while running the Copper Canyon trails. So when you're in the middle of the program, just think, you're building Tarahumara strength.

Upper-body and Core Strength

Enough of this picnic table at the bottom of Snow King Resort. Those slopes have been staring at us, begging us to give them some attention. We won't go too far. The altitude and the steep, endless incline will wreak some havoc—and quickly.

Ready. Go . . .

Hey, pretty good running. Knowledge is power, they say, and maybe you've got an extra bounce in your step now that you have a better grasp of how the body should operate as you use it. Feel those feet, how they strike the slope. Even if you're wearing shoes, run like you're not, like your bare feet are hitting the trail with each stride. Feel the firing in your calves. Be aware of your glutes and quads. Are they working? How hard? Amazing how quickly we feel the burn during a steep climb.

Okay, keep it going, but now focus on your core and upper body. Notice how your arms help drive your legs. Pump them higher; feel how your legs lift as well. It's almost like you're a marionette, your hands connected to your opposite knees by a string.

The farther we go up, the more I want you to be mindful of what is happening above your waist. Sense how you're working your core and upper body. As you tire—and you will tire on this bear of a mountain—notice changes in your form. Are you slumping over, shoulders rolled, stomach collapsed, struggling for breath? Or, though you feel some burn in your legs, is your back still straight, like a plank of wood, shoulders square, stomach tight, still drawing in deep breaths, easy and, most important, relaxed? Can I guess? Regardless, the difference has much to do with the strength of our core and upper body.

When we talk strength there, our aim is no different than with our feet and legs. We want endurance, stability, power, mobility, and that all too important muscle equilibrium. If you want big pecs, no neck, and Popeye biceps, you'll fit right in at Venice Beach, California. But here in Jackson, you'll stand out—and catch a few snickers from folks. Given the mania here for adventure sports, most of us know what true strength looks like. Remember those climbers at the bouldering park below. As I said, that's the ideal of athleticism.

Slow down and stop now. Grab your knees if you need to and take a few deep breaths. Here, have a sip from my water bottle and take a long look around you: nothing but mountains and sky in every direction. See the Grand Tetons over there at thirteen thousand–plus feet? You will be exploring those mountains soon.

When we develop strength in the core and upper body, we do ourselves a world of good for our running. We swing our arms better and move with greater mobility. We activate muscles along the spine that protect the whole body, allowing us to run upright with greater stabilization. We breathe easier. We run more relaxed. We maintain form economy better and longer, especially during those last few miles when everything feels like it wants to collapse.

In the alternative, if we fail to pursue whole-body strength, trouble ensues. Interconnectedness gives as much as it takes. Almost as a rule, runners tend to get rounded shoulders, thereby tightening our pectorals, thereby pulling on the muscles in our back, which causes pain while running—and, let's be frank, in everyday life as well. These same rounded shoulders affect our breathing and the mobility of our arms and upper body. Without mobility there, our torso moves side to side as we run. This throws off our efficiency and equilibrium, and as we tire—more quickly, by the way—we begin to lean over our feet or hunch.

The same occurs if our core, particularly our abdominals and the muscles in our lower back, are weak or not firing properly. During a long run, have you ever experienced an annoying pain between the shoulder blades and spine, or felt your back muscles kind of catch with each breath or begin to ache? If your answer is yes, you have some work to do on your upper body and core. Don't worry; we all do.

In many ways, this training will resemble the same kind of movements that climbers use when they go up a cliff face or navigate a boulder park. There's lots of back-and-forth, side-to-side, and three-dimensional movements. You'll be holding some muscles in position for a prolonged time (clinically referred to as isometric), while other parts of your body are moving. Think of a climber holding a cliff wall with two hands while he is swinging his lower body across to find a new toehold.

In running, like climbing, you want to promote a body that mobilizes and stabilizes at the same time in different parts of the body. Through exercises with a Fitball, you'll do exactly that.

I know you're anxious—and a little fearful—to get cracking on the exercise program now that I've won you over to the idea of strength and muscle equilibrium throughout the body. Be patient—plenty of time for you to fire muscles that you didn't even know existed. On the way down the slope, we'll touch on the importance of awareness as we execute the program.

Awareness and Strength Training

If a free climber allows his mind to wander, loses form, and executes a wrong move, he faces big trouble—the long, backbreaking kind. As runners, we face much less severe consequences for a lack of awareness. That said, if we want to reap the tremendous advantages that come with strength training, we must concentrate, keeping our senses attuned throughout the program.

The good thing is that the exercises I've developed will also improve your level of awareness. While you do the slant board exercises, you will be forced to know how you are using your big toe, arch, and the rest of your foot. In other exercises, as you stabilize some parts of your body while moving others, you can't help but be very mindful of how your body is acting, reacting, where you feel tense, where loose.

Many of the exercises require close attention to form. They ask you to perform movements that you can't see yourself, demanding you to feel your body, visualize what it's doing, thereby creating an awareness of how your body is moving. This creates an understanding of how your body moves, and how it needs to relax to operate powerfully and efficiently. When you have to mentally and physically work hard at the same time to execute an exercise, great results ensue.

Not only will you develop more strength with this mindfulness, but as you train, you are also developing muscle memory. The more exercises you do over time, the more your muscles will know on a subconscious level what to do and how they should be used in equilibrium. They'll understand what feels good and right without your even thinking about it.

Awareness drives performance, and if you remain mindful through the strength program, you'll see great results, particularly as you begin working on run form.

TRUE STRENGTH PROGRAM

Exercise Philosophy

Think of yourself as a martial artist. Be aware; work to get the movements of these exercises correct. Allow me to repeat: Awareness and form are preeminent, and besides working through this program barefoot (and sockless), they are the only rules. Stay true to these rules and you will develop true strength over time. There's no use counting reps if you lose form halfway through your set. More is not always better. Better is better. Take a second, take in that statement again, and understand it. Better is better. Do the work to get these exercises right.

As an athlete and coach, I know most people's instinct with this program will be to hammer through each exercise, the entire list, with each workout. Get out of that mind-set. A commitment to this program is the key. Do what you can, when you can, but keep at it. Since we are working for equilibrium, hitting both the big dominant and supporting muscles, you can perform these exercises frequently—unlike more traditional strength training. Yes, in the beginning, you might find yourself sore and in need of a few days off, but this will pass.

Staying consistent means trying to do at least a little every day. I know your life is busy. But the beauty of this program is that it's not only okay, but encouraged, to do some of this circuit every day. Sometimes focus on one or two exercises, if that's what your schedule permits. Then, when a window opens, do the whole circuit. Also, try to do some of the slant board exercises right before a run. The exercises will activate your muscles, giving you a "good feel" for form before you hit the trail. We're not talking an hour of strength training before a twenty-miler. A little bit goes a long way. Same goes for common sense.

When you begin these exercises, take them slowly; don't work past your level of ability. I've designed the program as a progression. Some at the end of the program you will not be able to do initially. That's okay. Use some patience and put your ego in check. Again, work like a martial artist: deliberate movement and consistent practice. Through these exercises, you will improve, you will develop new strength where you need it, you will grow stronger than you ever imagined, and you will create muscle memory that will help you as you work on run form.

Also get creative. Keep it fresh. I'll give you pointers on how to challenge yourself, but don't depend on me. Mix up the number of reps you do (eight, ten, twelve, or sets of two or three) and vary the lengths of a set (how many exercises you are doing), the speed with which you do each move, and even the location where you execute these exercises. Take it to the track or the park. Work it while listening to music in the living room. Have fun.

One last point—and keep reminding yourself of this whenever you do these exercises: This program, both the foot/leg and upper body/core, is not meant to make you better at strength training for its own sake. Your goal here is to improve your athleticism, to train your body to work in harmonious sync, balanced and strong, so that you are a better, more natural runner. Form and awareness will get you there.

Equipment

To work through this program, you'll need a few pieces of equipment. Here's a brief guide to why I use each—and what kind you should buy (or look for at your gym). None of these will break the bank, but they're important to have on hand before you begin.

1. Slant Board

This single piece of equipment has opened up a whole new world to me. At first, you might be skeptical. A ramp of wood? How can that help? And these exercises, they look too easy. One of my athletes called them "fluffy" . . . until he began doing them. Like my other athletes, he felt right away how the slant board engaged his foot, particularly the big toe. Using various angles of the foot on the board, he activated his muscles all the way up to the hip. You'll be no different. A couple weeks into using the slant board, you'll be developing bomber foot strength and essential stability. These exercises are simple, potent, and usable every day.

Now, I have had custom-designed portable slant boards made for me, which are sized to fit only your forefoot and have a unique piece of wood on the ramp bottom that creates a performance-enhancing wobble effect. Check it out at www.runningwitheric.com. I know you will really dig the unique challenges it provides. That said, you'll find various slant boards online and at most gyms (typically used to stretch your calves) that will adequately get the job done. They come in all shapes and sizes, so just make sure the one you purchase looks something like my own.

2. Stability Disk

Beginning with the slant board, you'll move away from doing exercises flat-footed. Instead you'll execute them on your forefoot, heel elevated, mimicking your landing in running. Once you start to develop some foot strength with the slant board, you'll progress to the round stability disk. It adds more movement under your forefoot and will therefore push you to develop your muscle equilibrium even further. This harmless-looking little disk will fire a ton of muscle fibers and build incredible strength, without heavy weights and without adding bulk.

As with the slant board, my custom-made disks are perfect for these single-foot exercises and easy to take anywhere. Again, check it out at www.runningwitheric.com. That said, you'll find stability disks at your gym and at most good online fitness retailers that you can use for these exercises. Again, they come in various forms and go by different names (wobble board, for one), so check against my own to make sure you're getting the right kind of disk.

3. Fitball

We've all seen these large resistant stability balls that originated in Switzerland (and, therefore, go by the name "Swiss ball"). At first, they were used to help patients with cerebral palsy. Doctors, then physical therapists, and now coaches, trainers, and athletes have since found them to be of tremendous use for a variety of exercises. As opposed to working on a flat, stable surface, the Fitball requires you to maintain your balance, which fires more muscles—typically the smaller, more supportive ones that we need for core muscle equilibrium. You'll find Fitballs at almost every gym or sports store. Be sure to look at the height chart on the box (or online point of sale) to buy the right size Fitball for your body.

4. Ski Poles

Yes, you got it: ski poles—though walking sticks or a cutoff broom handle will also do. Not much to explain here other than that these are critical for maintaining position/form as you first develop your foot/leg strength. And just think, you'll get more use out of that expensive ski gear.

True Strength Program for the Foot/Leg/Glute

A. Slant Board Balance Sequence

We focus first on foot strength, laying the foundation. These exercises give you a feeling for how your foot reacts to the stability and strength required to stand on your forefoot, heel raised. As you develop, these exercises will stabilize and equalize your muscles all the way up the leg.

GENERAL INSTRUCTION

- Perform the slant board sequence three to five times per week.
- The three exercises below are a progression. They are not meant to be done together. One should be mastered before moving on to the second.
- Perfect for a prerun workout to activate the muscles in your legs.
- Always work barefoot and sockless.
- Focus on using your big toe for stability and balance.
- Hold poles perpendicular to the floor. The looser your grip, the better.
- If possible, work in front of a mirror.

- There are three positions of your foot on the board for each of these exercises:
    - uphill (big toe parallel and closest to top of the ramp)
    - downhill (big toe parallel and farthest from top of the ramp)
    - forward (big toe perpendicular and closest to top of the ramp).

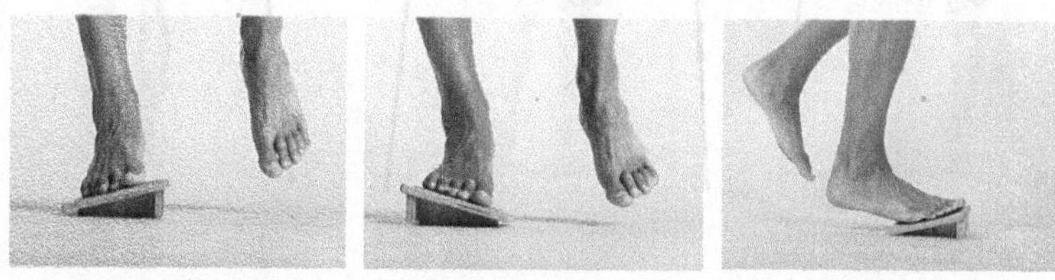

Uphill *Downhill* *Forward*

1. TWO-POLE BALANCE

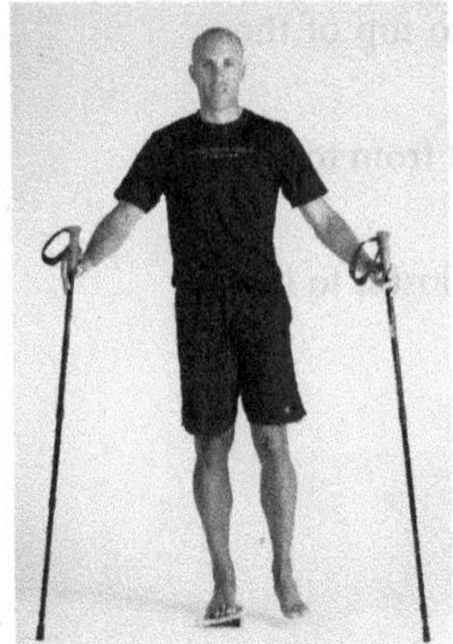
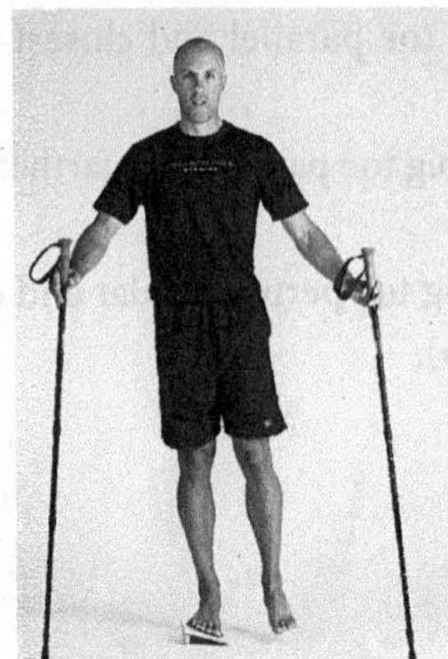
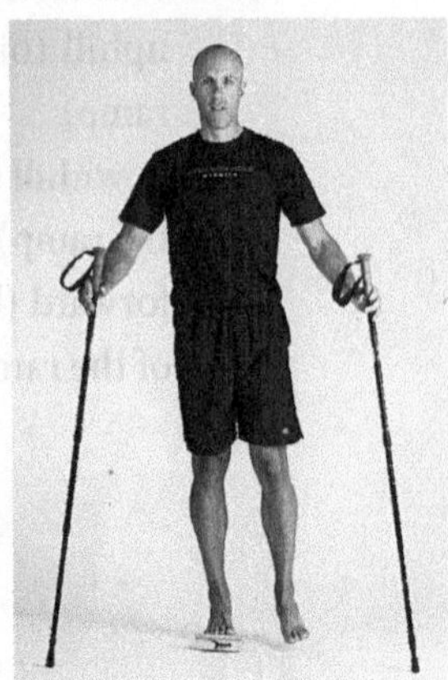

To perform, step on slant board with your right forefoot, arch and heel elevated, as you're able. Balance with your leg straight, knee locked, to activate the glute, and maintain this position as long as you can for up to one to two minutes. Execute three slant board directions (uphill, downhill, forward), alternating each leg after each slant board direction balance.

- Use poles to help you balance, but not as a crutch. Do not bend over or lean on them.
- Once you feel the two-pole balance is easy for two minutes (with arch/heel elevated, no excessive knee bend), you're ready to execute with a single pole.

2. ONE-POLE BALANCE

To perform, do the same actions as two-pole balance, but use only one pole to steady yourself. With one pole, you begin to sense how challenging this can be. Execute three slant board directions (uphill, downhill, forward), alternating each foot after each direction.

- Now that you have one pole, you can fight for your balance with your muscles a bit more. You don't need to be as concerned about having an upright body and straight leg.
- Switch which hand holds the pole to work your stability in different ways.
- Once you feel the one-pole balance is easy for two minutes (with arch/heel elevated, no excessive knee bend), you're ready to execute without poles.

3. NO POLE BALANCE

This is a very challenging exercise. To perform, do this the same way as previous exercises but without a pole. Balance as long as you can (up to a minute), three to five times on each foot, before switching slant board directions. Execute three slant board directions (uphill, downhill, forward), alternating each foot after each direction.

- Unlike the first two exercises, in slant board balance with no poles your body will move and contort. Have fun with it and fight for balance.
- Focus on balancing with your feet, not your body. Try to make your movements and contortions slow, and use your arms to help. Avoid quick jerking movements. Be relaxed.

B. Slant Board Movement Sequence

In the next set of exercises, we continue to work foot strength, but now we're adding some movement, which will increase the challenge for your calves, quads, and glutes—definitely a stability challenge, and it helps develop great run economy and form.

GENERAL INSTRUCTIONS

- Start this set of exercises at the same time you start the slant board balance sequence.
- Use as workout circuit, executing one after the next, three to five times per week.
- Perfect for a prerun workout to activate the muscles in your legs.
- Always work barefoot and sockless.
- Focus on using your big toe for stability and balance.
- Hold poles perpendicular to the floor. The looser your grip, the better. Use your poles—they are your friends—but do not lean on them.
- If possible, work in front of a mirror.
- Unlike balance sequence, each exercise has only a single slant board direction.
- We are working the muscles of the leg on the slant board (board leg), not the leg that moves (nonboard leg).
- With this exercise, it's very important to keep the board leg straight. Lock it out.

1. SIDE LIFT

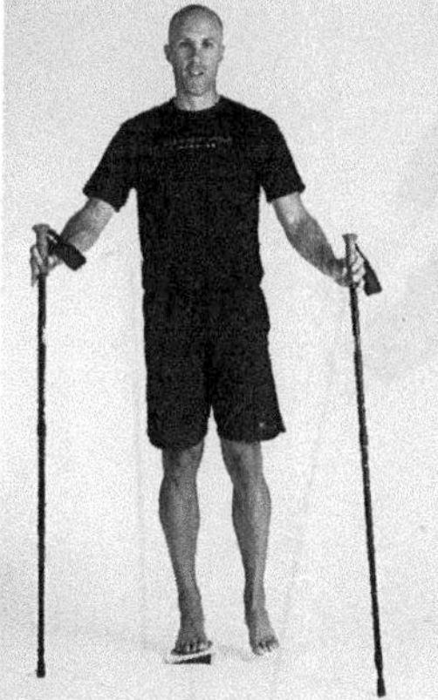

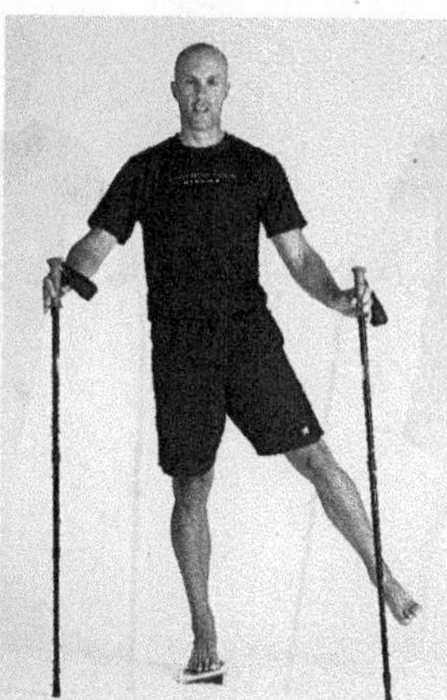

To perform, start with your right foot, stepping on the slant board in an uphill position, arch and heel elevated, as you're able. Now, balance on the right foot with your right leg (board leg) straight, knee locked. Keep left leg (nonboard leg) straight too, and the left foot off the floor. Keeping your left leg straight, move it out to the side, away from your right leg. Pause at the top of the range of motion for one to two seconds; then bring the left leg back down to start position.

- The sideways movement should be smooth, fluid, controlled. You are not looking for an excessive range of motion or speed. This is not a stretch.
- Keep the nonboard leg's toes/foot straight ahead at all times.
- Hips should remain level and even during this leg movement.
- This slant position helps create mobility/flexibility for those with high arches.
- Progress to doing twenty to twenty-five repetitions (reps) with each leg. Work only to your current ability, while maintaining an elevated heel and straight leg.

2. FROG LIFT

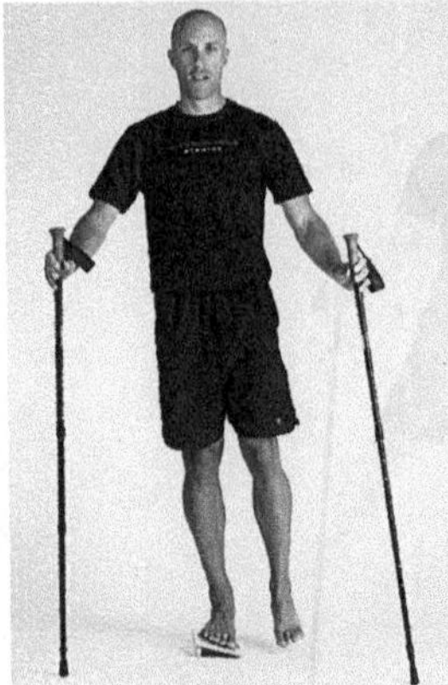
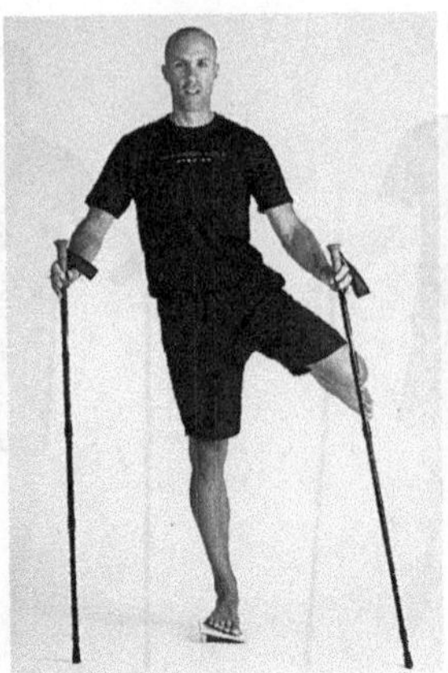
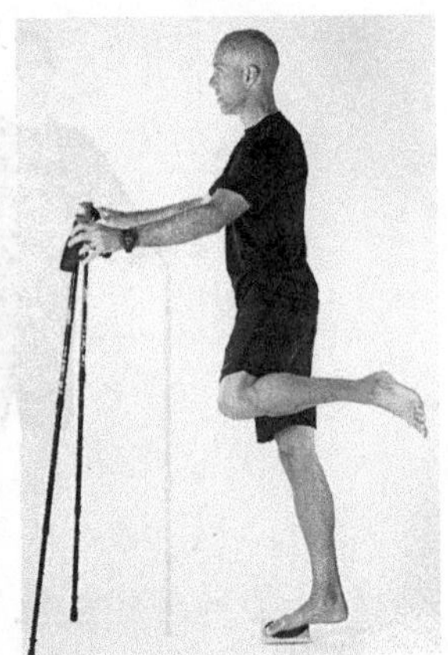

To perform, start with your right foot, stepping on the slant board in a downhill position, arch and heel elevated, as you're able. Balance on the right foot with your right leg (board leg) straight, knee locked. Keep left leg (nonboard leg) straight too, and the left foot off the floor. Then, with your left leg, make a bend at the knee as you simultaneously lift it away from your right leg. Pause at the top of the range of motion for one to two seconds with your ankle height level with your knee; then bring the left leg back down to start position.

- We are conducting a side lift, but it's a bent-knee one (not straight leg, as in the previous exercise). Your left leg should be bent at a ninety-degree angle, and your ankle should be at a height level with your knee.
- The movement should be smooth, fluid, controlled. You are not looking for an excessive range of motion or speed. This is not a stretch.
- Hips should remain level and even during this leg movement.
- This slant position will be good for runners with a flat foot, as it will strengthen the arch.
- Progress to doing twenty to twenty-five reps with each leg. Work only to your current ability, but maintain an elevated heel and straight leg.

3. KNEE DRIVE

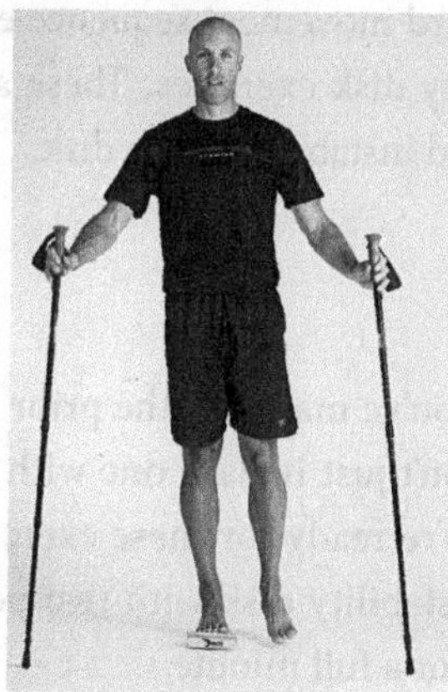
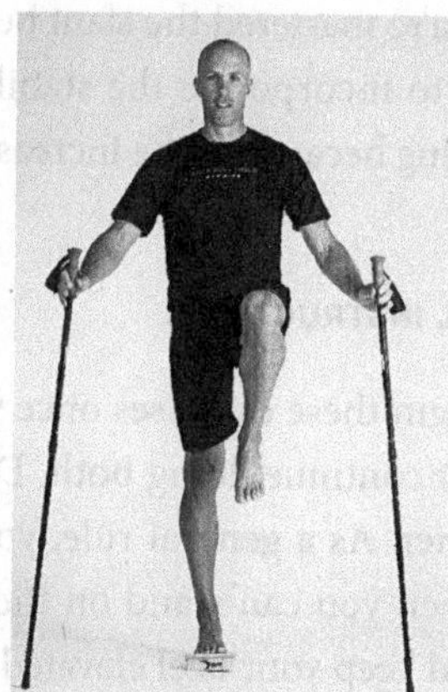

To perform, start with your right foot, stepping on the slant board in a forward position, arch and heel elevated, as you're able. Balance on the right foot with your right leg (board leg) straight, knee locked. Keep left leg (nonboard leg) straight too, and the left foot off the floor. Then, with your left leg, lift your knee as high as you can toward your chest, while keeping your left ankle and heel under your hamstring, and your right leg straight and locked out. Pause at the top of the range of motion for one to two seconds, feeling the board leg's glute activate; then bring the left leg back down to start position.

- This exercise helps to increase your stride length—improving speed, power, and economy.
- Progress to doing twenty to twenty-five reps with each leg. Work only to your current ability, but maintain an elevated heel and straight leg.

C. Stability Disk Movement Sequence

Once you're mastered the slant board movement sequence exercises, it's time to incorporate the stability disk exercises. These are more challenging because of the increased instability of the disk.

GENERAL INSTRUCTIONS

- Begin these exercises once you've mastered the prior set, but continue doing both. Don't just replace one with the other. As a general rule, you're ready for these exercises when you can stand on the stability disk with two poles and keep your heel elevated for a full minute.
- Use as a workout circuit, executing one after the next, two to three times per week.
- Perfect for a prerun workout to activate the muscles in your legs.
- Always work barefoot and sockless.
- Focus on using your entire forefoot and toes for stability and balance.
- Hold poles perpendicular to the floor. The looser your grip, the better. Use your poles—they are your friends—but do not lean on them.
- If possible, work in front of a mirror.
- We are working the muscles of the leg on the stability disk (disk leg), not the leg that moves (nondisk leg).
- With this exercise, it's very important to keep the disk leg straight. Lock it out.

1. SIDE LIFT

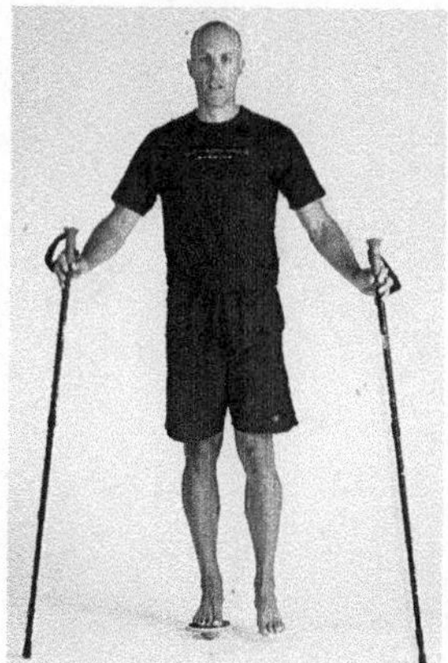

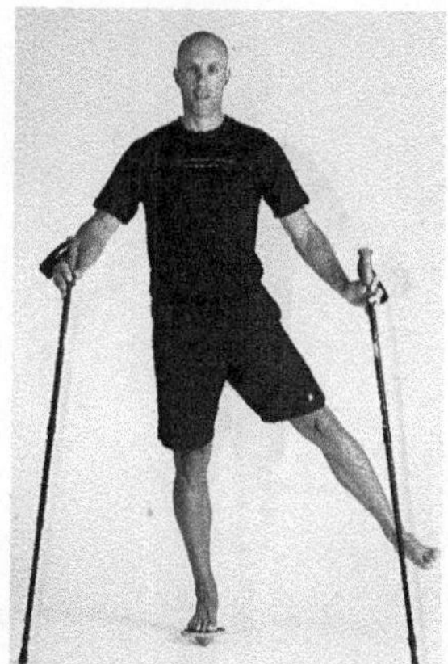

To perform, start with your right foot, stepping on the stability disk, arch and heel elevated, as you're able. Balance on the right foot with your right leg (disk leg) straight, knee locked. Keep left leg (nondisk leg) straight too, and the left foot off the floor. Keeping your left leg straight, move it out to the side, away from your right leg. Pause at the top of the range of motion for one to two seconds; then bring the left leg back down to start position.

- The sideways movement should be smooth, fluid, controlled. You are not looking for an excessive range of motion or speed. This is not a stretch.
- Keep the nondisk leg's toes/foot straight ahead at all times.
- Hips should remain level and even during this leg movement.
- Progress to doing twenty to twenty-five reps with each leg. Work only to your current ability, but maintain an elevated heel and straight leg.

2. KNEE DRIVE

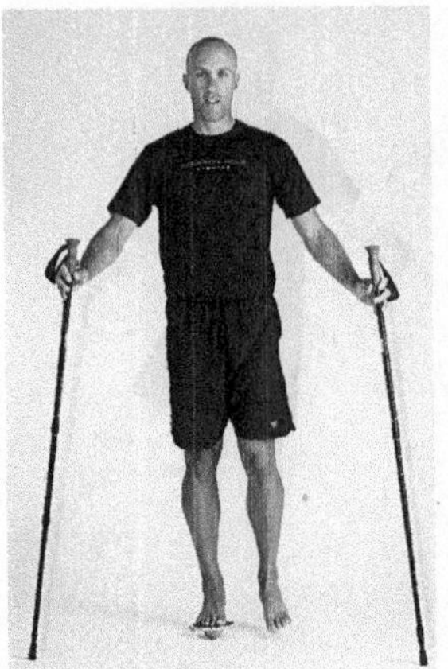
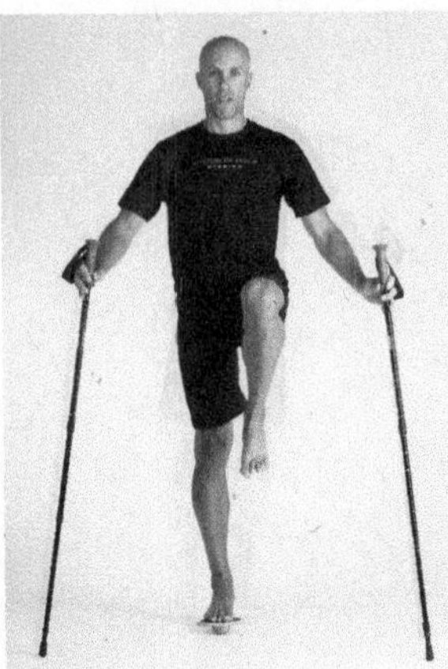

To perform, start with your right foot, stepping on the stability disk in a forward position, arch and heel elevated, as you're able. Balance on the right foot with your right leg (board leg) straight, knee locked. Keep left leg (nonboard leg) straight too, and the left foot off the floor. Then, with your left leg, lift your knee as high as you can toward your chest, while keeping your left ankle and heel under your hamstring, and your right leg straight and locked out. Pause at the top of the range of motion for one to two seconds, feeling the board leg's glute activate; then bring the left leg back down to start.

- Progress to doing twenty to twenty-five reps with each leg. Work only to your current ability, but maintain an elevated heel and straight leg.

D. Dynamic Leg Strength, Stability, and Power

The next exercises are different because they are executed with a lot of movement, which really develops speed and power.

GENERAL INSTRUCTIONS

- Use as a workout circuit, executing one after the next, two to three times per week.
- Except for the flat-footed Fitball lunge, you aren't ready for these exercises until you can stand on the stability disk with two poles and keep your heel elevated for a full minute.
- Always work barefoot and sockless.
- Focus on using your entire forefoot and toes for stability and balance.
- Hold poles perpendicular to the floor. The looser your grip, the better. Use your poles—they are your friends—but do not lean on them.
- If possible, work in front of a mirror.

1. FITBALL LUNGE SEQUENCE—FLAT FOOT/SLANT BOARD/DISK

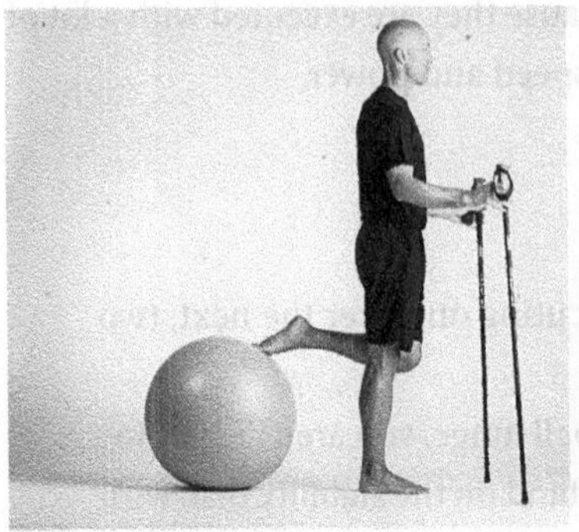

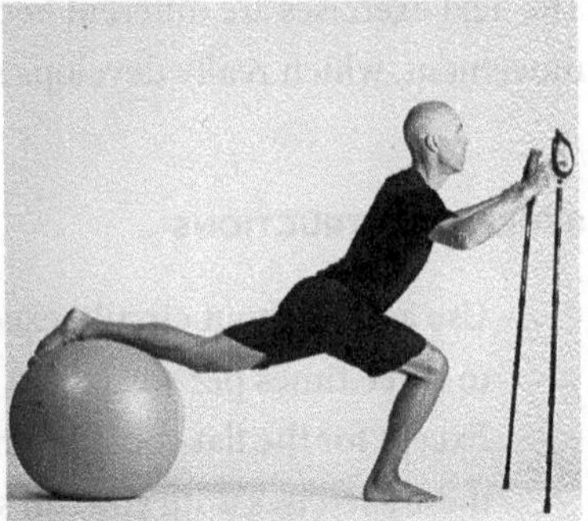

To perform the basic flat-foot exercise, stand straight on your right leg flat-footed. This will be your lunge leg. The foot of your left leg, which is your ball leg, should be raised up behind you and resting on top of the Fitball. Using the poles for balance, squat down as far as your range of motion will allow, while moving the ball leg back, rolling the Fitball with it. Return to starting position.

- This is one exercise, with three progressions. You'll do it first with your foot flat on the floor. Once you master that, you'll move on to doing it on a slant board. Once you've got that down, you'll do it on the stability disk.
- The objective is to keep as much weight as you can on the lunge leg and as little weight as possible on the ball leg.
- If the Fitball scoots out to the side, this means your hips are moving and unstable. Don't be beleaguered. This is exactly why we're working this exercise. Keep to form so you work those muscles right, and keep your hips level. Over time you'll develop the muscle memory and strength to make it happen.
- Your focus should be on moving the ball leg straight back, which allows the lunge to take place. This also increases the range of motion and adds mobility challenges.
- Avoid moving the lunge leg's knee forward and back; focus on just moving the knee up and down. If there is too much

forward and backward movement, there's too much weight on the back leg on the ball.

- Your goal is to do three sets, gradually working your way up to twenty to twenty-five reps with each leg.
- Progression advice: Once you're able to do three sets, twenty to twenty-five reps on each leg, flat-footed, then progress to slant board. Your lunge-leg foot should be on the slant board in *uphill position only*. As with other slant board exercises, keep your arch and heel elevated. Progress to doing three sets of twenty to twenty-five reps with each leg. Once you progress to the slant board, you don't have to continue performing this exercise flat-footed.

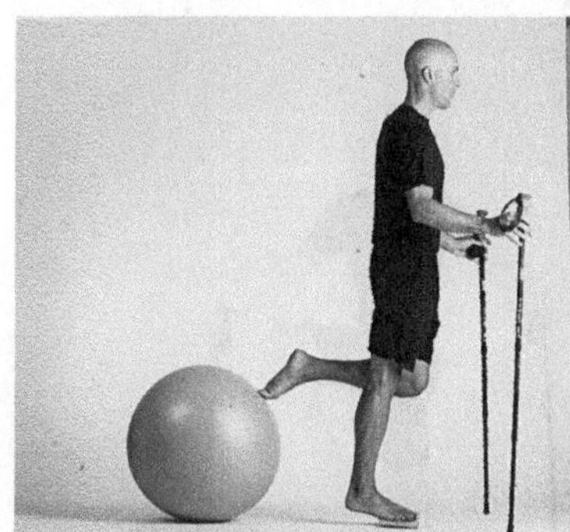
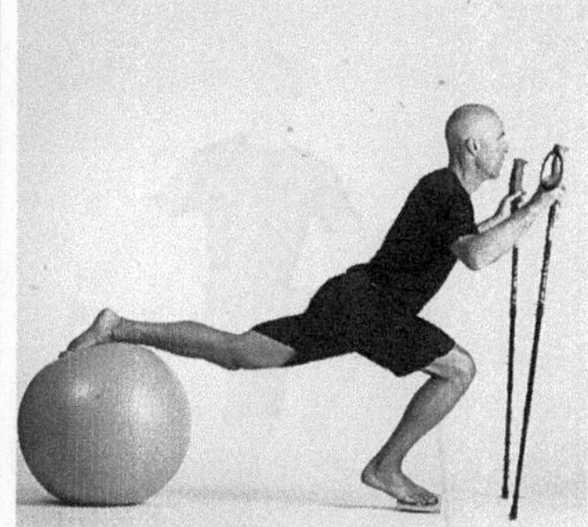

- Once you're able to do three sets, twenty to twenty-five reps, on the slant board, you're ready for the stability disk. Once you progress to the stability disk, you don't have to continue performing this exercise on the slant board.

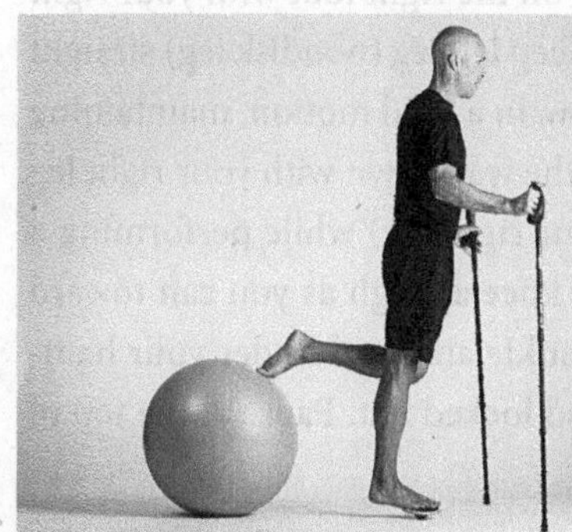
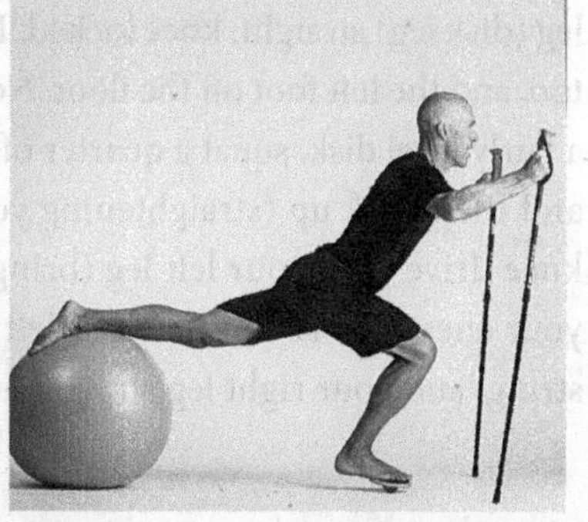

2. RUN SQUAT WITH ROTATIONS

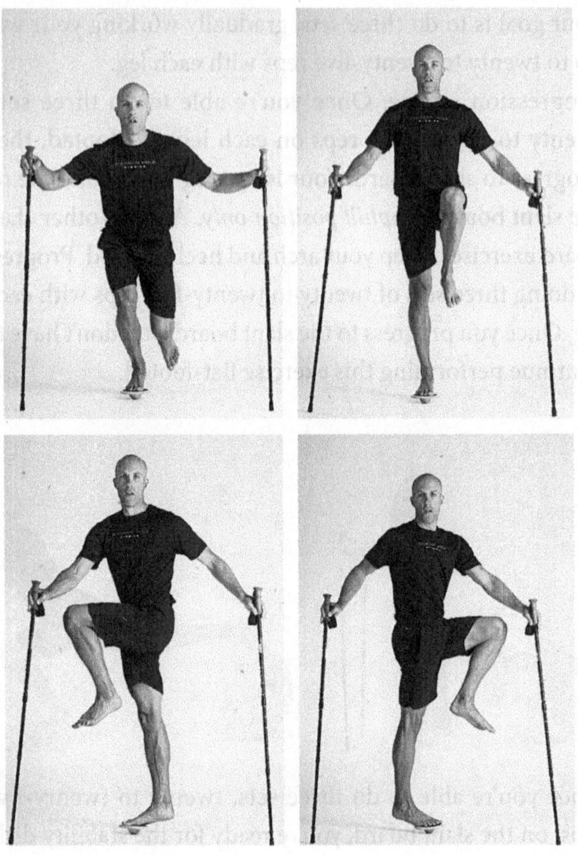

To perform, start with your right foot, stepping on the disk, arch and heel elevated, as you're able. Balance on the right foot with your right leg (disk leg) straight, knee locked. Keep left leg (nondisk leg) straight too, and the left foot off the floor. Now, in a fluid motion, maintaining a fairly level disk, squat a quarter of the way down with your right leg and then back up (straightening your right leg) while performing a knee drive with your left leg (bring knee as high as you can toward your chest). Note to keep your left ankle and heel under your hamstring, and your right leg straight and locked out. Pause at the top of the range of motion for one to two seconds, feeling the disk leg's glute activate. Then rotate as far as you can to each side while keeping your shoulders square and your knee high. Keep your eyes straight ahead the whole time. Then bring the left leg back down to start position.

- This is a complicated exercise, and when you're first starting it, you shouldn't try to do it all at once. Instead, break down the movements and do them one at a time. Take them slowly and get the form right. Once you've got each step down, then put it all together and concentrate on executing it fluidly.
- We are working the disk leg. Remember to keep it straight when rotating the body side to side.
- Your goal is to do three sets. Gradually work your way up to eight to twelve reps with each leg. Work only to your current ability while maintaining an elevated heel and straight leg.

3. ONE-LEG PISTOL SQUATS

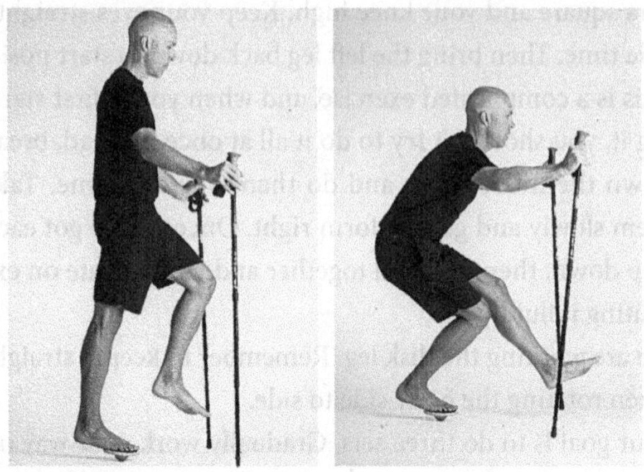

To perform, start with your right foot, stepping on the stability disk, arch and heel elevated, as you're able. Next, squat down on your right leg as far as your range of motion will allow while maintaining a fairly level disk. Keep your left leg out in front of you at all times, kind of in Karate Kid stance. Then come up from your squat, with your right leg locked. Pause for one to two seconds; feel your glute activate.

- Squat like you're sitting down in a chair. Fold your chest forward (work with your body). Avoid moving the squat leg's knee forward and tipping the disk toward its front edge.
- At the beginning, you don't need a big range of motion. Just do what you can, and build up to a full squat with time.
- As you improve, add some speed and try to rise up with a powerful explosion to your movement.
- Your goal is to do three sets. Gradually work your way up to twenty to twenty-five reps with each leg. Work only to your current ability while maintaining an elevated heel and straight leg.

Performing Your Circuit and Progressions

You want to try to perform the complete circuit up to two to three times per week, with one to two days off between. When you have time to do a complete circuit, here's how it should work: Follow each exercise block (A, B, C, D) in order, but following the progressions we described. In other words, if you're just beginning, you should do exercise blocks A, B, and D (but only Fitball lunge flat-footed). Once you're able to move on to the stability disk, then you can do all the exercise blocks (A, B, C, D), and all the exercises within each sequence.

Follow the circuit in this order, introducing progressions (*) when you are ready:

A. Slant board balance sequence:
   1. Double-pole balance
   2. Single-pole balance (*)
   3. No-pole balance (*)

B. Slant board movement sequence:
   1. Side lift
   2. Frog lift
   3. Knee drive

C. Stability disk movement sequence (*):
   1. Side lift (*)
   2. Knee drive (*)

D. Dynamic leg strength, stability, and power:
   1. Fitball lunge sequence
      - Flat foot
      - Slant board (*)
      - Disk (*)
   2. Run squat with rotations (*)
   3. One-Leg Pistol Squats

Strength Program for the Upper Body/Core

Introductory Fitball Exercise Progressions

This Fitball regimen trains full-body movements, not just muscles, and will strengthen your core and upper body, stimulate your nervous system, and maximize your running ability.

1. KNEES TO CHEST

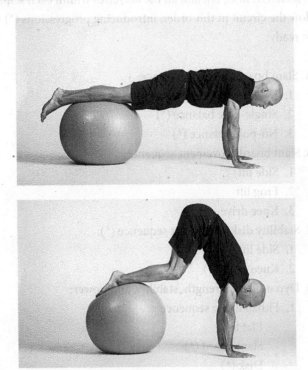

To perform, assume a plank position, placing your legs on top of the ball and your arms in a push-up position, elbows locked. Then roll the Fitball toward your arms while pulling your knees to your chest (thus the clever name). As you bring your knees to your chest, lift your glutes upward. Return to plank, engaging stomach in between reps. Repeat.

- While you execute this exercise, be careful to keep your toes pointed out and avoid bending your elbows excessively.
- No rocking back and forth with shoulders (fore and aft), and keep your back from sagging.
- As a beginner, you can keep the ball closer to your knees to start, and as you progress, move the ball toward your feet to increase difficulty.
- In this exercise, we fire a lot of the core. Our goal here is to work on stabilization and strength endurance throughout our upper back and shoulders.
- Your goal is to do this ten to twenty reps. Always work to your ability.

2. WINDSHIELD WIPERS

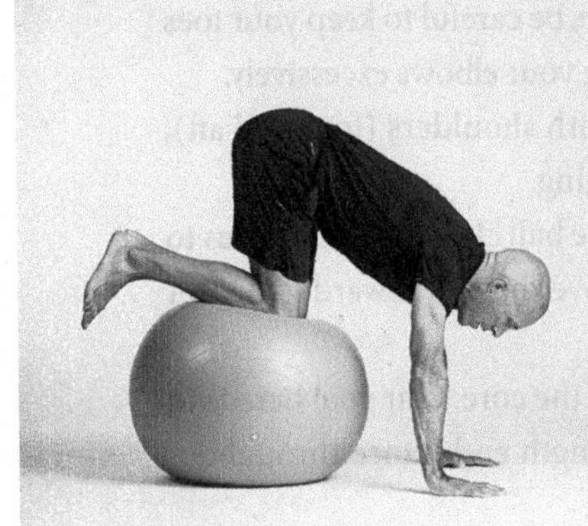

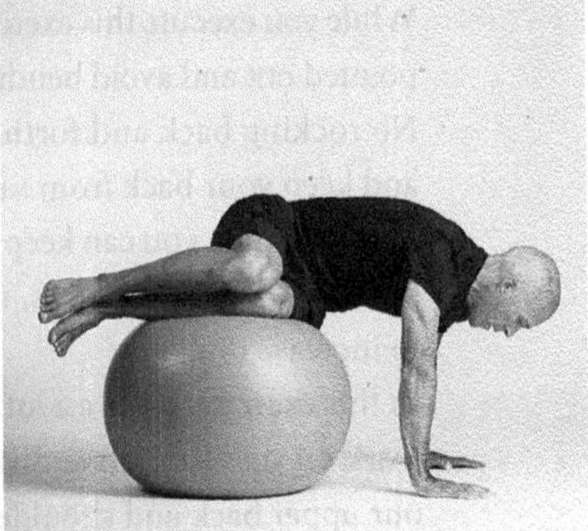

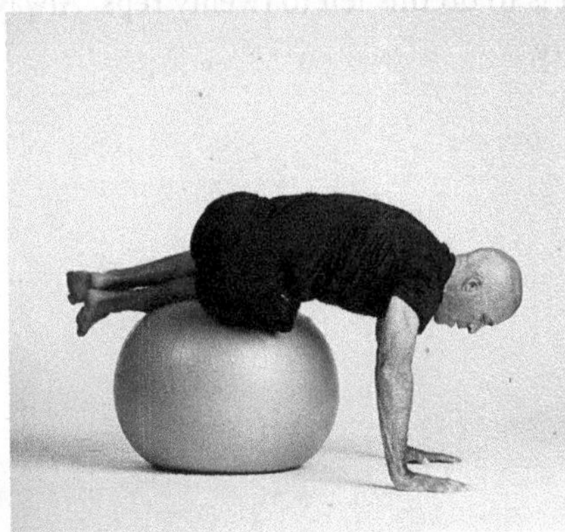

To perform, start with your knees on top of the Fitball, your arms shoulder width apart, and your hands on the floor. Now rotate your hips from side to side, keeping your knees bent. Initiate and control your movement and rotation with your abdominals.

- For stability, keep your palms flat on the floor and your fingers spread wide.
- Maintain your knees bent at a ninety-degree angle on top of the ball and drawn slightly toward chest.
- While you're doing this, keep your forearms as close as

possible to the ball. Don't let your elbows bend excessively, especially during rotation.

- Work on increasing range of motion first and then add a bit of speed.
- In this exercise, we train our hips to rotate, which often runners are unable to do fluidly because of tightness in the hip flexors and lower back. We're also firing our stomachs during this exercise, allowing us to generate power through our abdomen, which we'll use when we're running.
- Your goal is to do this ten to twenty reps on each side. Work to your ability.

3. SCORPIONS

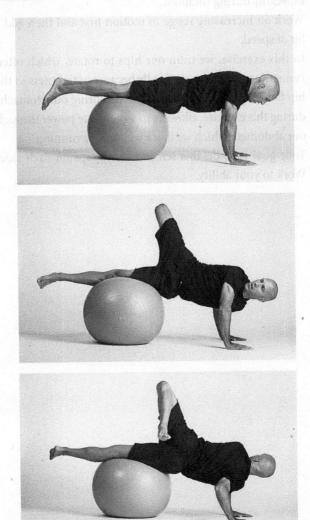

To perform, assume a plank position, Fitball between your hips and knees, and your arms in a push-up position, elbows locked. Rotate your hips to the left as you roll onto the side of the right leg. Keeping your right leg straight and stable, reach your left foot as close to your right elbow as possible. During this movement, keep your knee high and pointing toward the ceiling. Hold that position for one to two seconds. Then return to the plank position. Repeat on the other side of your body.

- This is a real twister, so be aware of how and where your body is moving throughout.
- Keep your ball leg straight and rigid. This is key to getting the movement right.
- Keep stomach tight and avoid sagging of the back.
- Allow the elbow of the arm opposite the moving leg to bend. That will increase your range of motion and activate the muscles in your upper back.
- In this exercise, we really work the chest, shoulders, and back, combating that hunched-over syndrome that throws off our natural stride. Performing this exercises creates a lot of mind/body awareness as you attempt to get the form right. The mobility and balance challenges of executing the Scorpion will foster your athleticism.
- Your goal is to do this eight to fifteen reps on each side. Work to your ability.
- To see a video demonstration of this exercise, visit runningwitheric.com.

4. ISO BRIDGE

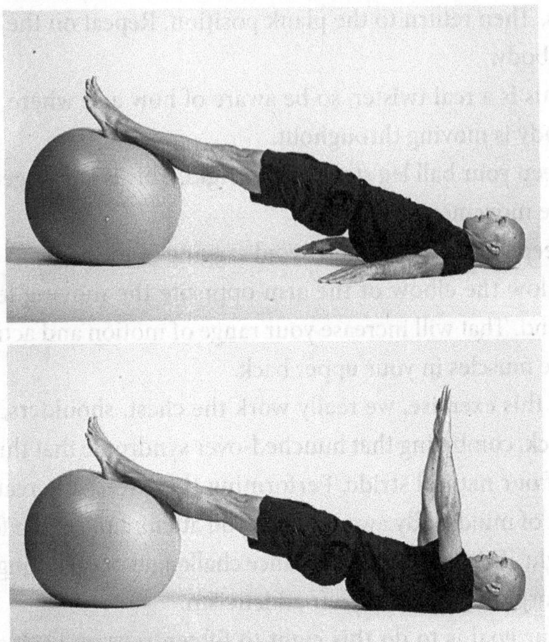

- To perform, start on your back with your shoulders and head on the floor, arms out to the sides, palms flat on the floor. Your feet should be on the top of the Fitball and your body in a straight line. Focus on lifting your hips, like someone's pulling a string upward from your sides. To increase the challenge, bring your arms straight above you. Hold that position as long as you can. Then return your hands to the ground.
- While you are doing this exercise, keep your focus on maintaining your hips high and your body in a straight line.
- Squeeze your glutes and keep your body rigid. Place your awareness on your lower back.
- Keep your feet side by side, pointed up. No duck feet.

- This exercise focuses on your lower back, glutes, and the stabilizing muscles of the spine. It also engages the hamstrings. Depending on the placement of your arms, you get two exercises in one here.
- Your goal is to maintain the position for one to two minutes. Don't try that the first time you do this. Work up to it.

5. KNEE TOGGLE

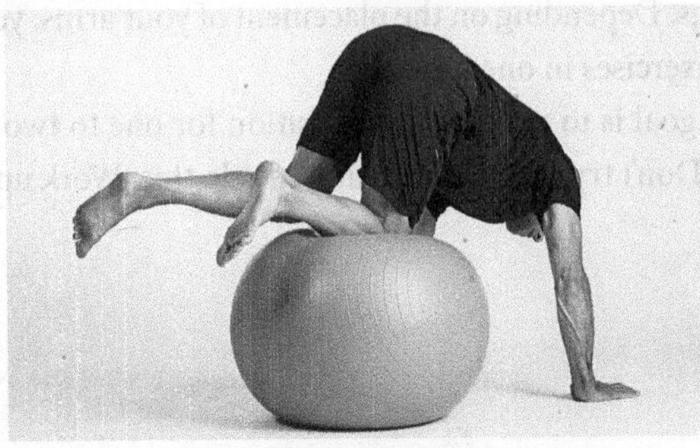

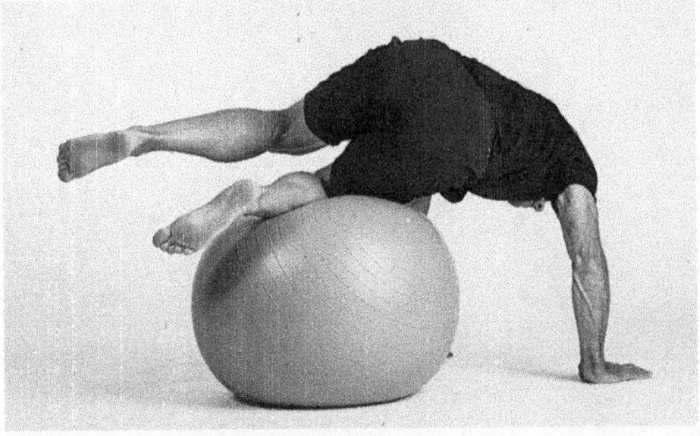

- To perform, kneel on the Fitball with your right knee. This leg is carrying the weight of your body. Your left leg should also be bent, but off the ball. Your hands should be shoulder width apart on the floor with the Fitball as close to your arms as possible at all times. Now rotate your hips to the left, allowing the ball to roll onto the side of your right leg, keeping your knee bent at ninety degrees. Then return to initial position. This is a continuous back-and-forth movement. Repeat on the other side, with your left leg on the ball and your right leg off it.
- The leg off the ball should remain bent, and don't let it rest on the working leg.
- To initiate the movement, use your hip/gluteus medius to rotate.

- To come back up from the side of your leg, focus on pushing into the ball with your knee.
- Keep your elbows and arms as straight as you can during rotation, and activate your abs the entire time to help control the movement.
- Despite its name, this is really a full-body challenge that will improve our athleticism and running. In these movements, we're creating power and stabilization in the glutes and the core.
- Your goal is to do this eight to fifteen reps for each leg. Work to your ability.
- To see a video demonstration of this exercise, visit runningwitheric.com.

6. FROG CRUNCH

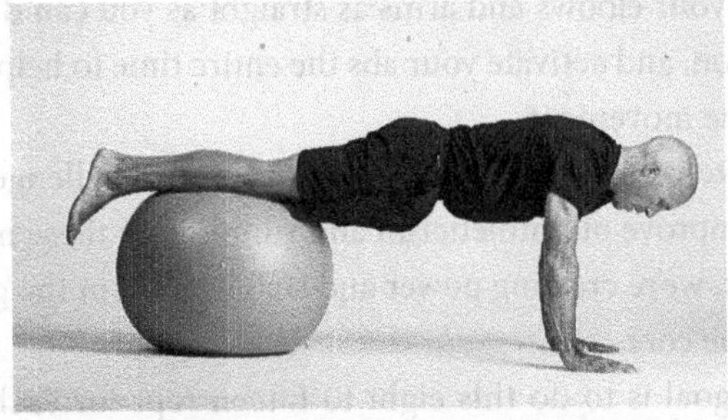

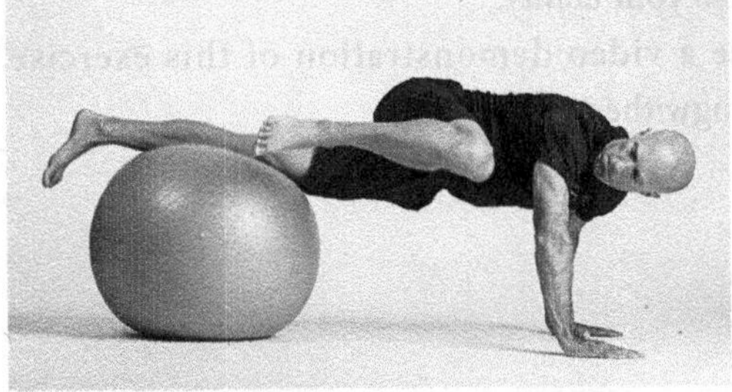

To perform, assume a plank position, placing your legs on top of the Fitball and your arms in a push-up position, elbows locked. Lift your right knee to your right elbow while rotating your head to look at your knee. Pause for one to two seconds and then return to a plank. Keep your left leg straight and rigid throughout this movement. Repeat with the same leg for a full set of reps. Then do a set of reps for the other leg. Once you get strong on this exercise, progress to alternating legs with each move.

- This is not a fast movement; don't throw your leg up there—control it.
- Keep your back straight and your stomach tight.
- As a beginner, you can keep the ball closer to your knees to start, and as you progress, move the ball toward your feet to increase difficulty.
- This exercise concentrates on the core, particularly activating, through rotation, the side abdominals.
- Your goal is to do eight to fifteen reps per leg. Work to your ability.

7. ROCKERS

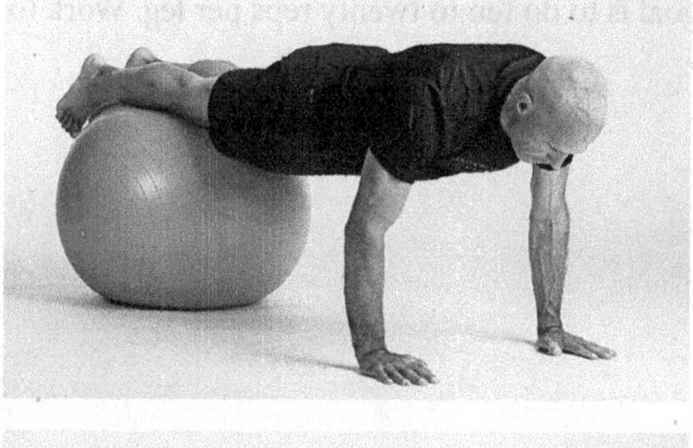

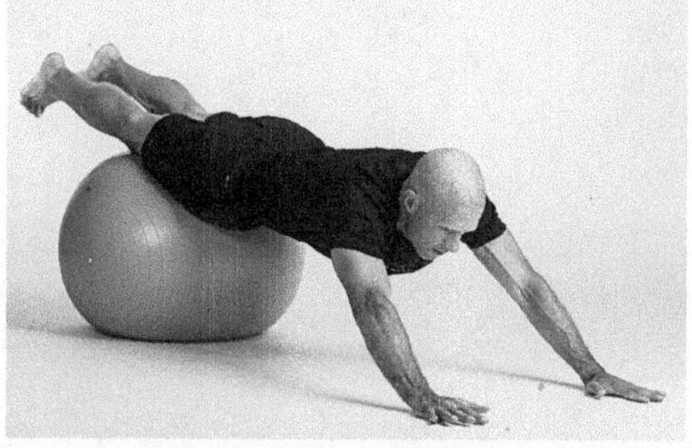

To perform, assume a plank position, placing your legs on top of the Fitball and your arms in a push-up position, elbows locked. Now, push yourself backward with your hands, slanting your upper body as you rock back on the ball, and allow your legs to go high in the air as you extend your reach, then return. Repeat.

- Keep your toes pointed and your legs and body straight and very rigid.
- If this hurts your lower back, move the ball closer to you (to make it easier); lift your hips and tighten your stomach. Don't let your back sag.
- As a beginner, you can keep the ball closer to your hips to start. As you progress, move the ball toward your feet to increase difficulty. Also, make the movement very slow and short to further challenge yourself.

- Similar to the previous exercise, the rocker really works the lower abs and your core, as well as promoting shoulder stability.
- Your goal is to do ten to twenty reps per leg. Work to your ability.

Advanced Fitball Exercise Progressions

Per the name, these are high-level progressions on exercises you've already done. Work yourself up to these movements only after you master exercises one through seven, above. Think like a martial artist, improving your athleticism step by step to get here.

1. JACKKNIFE (ADVANCED EXERCISE)

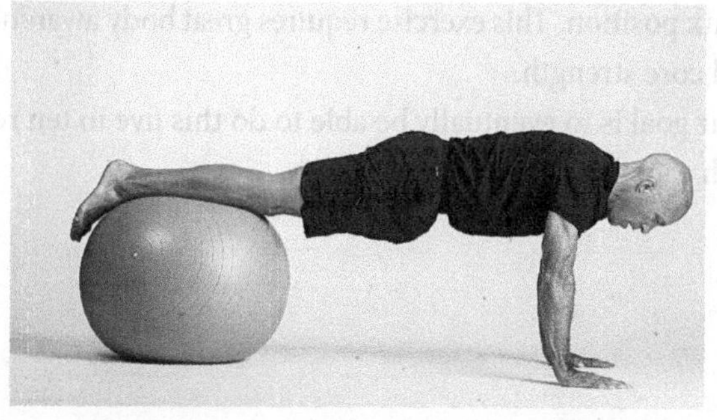

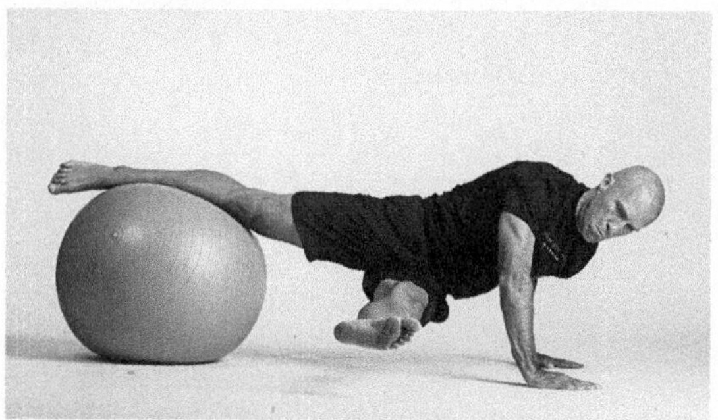

To perform, assume a plank position, placing your legs on top of the Fitball between your knees and ankles and your arms in a push-up position, elbows locked. Now bend your left leg and swing it underneath your body while rotating the left hip. Try to get your leg at a ninety-degree angle to your body. Return and repeat on the same side.

- Allow your elbows to bend to help you with the rotation.
- Ball placement should allow you to get your leg under you.

If you can't support the ball this far away from you, you are not ready to do this exercise yet. Keep working on frog crunch and rocker.

- If your back sags, you are not ready yet. Keep working on frog crunch and rocker.
- The jackknife is a bonanza of strength and stabilization for the upper body. You'll be hitting the abdominals and full upper body throughout this rotation. You'll also be stabilizing your shoulder through the tension of holding a plank position. This exercise requires great body awareness and core strength.
- Your goal is to eventually be able to do this five to ten reps with each leg. Work to your ability.

2. CAN OPENER (ADVANCED EXERCISE)

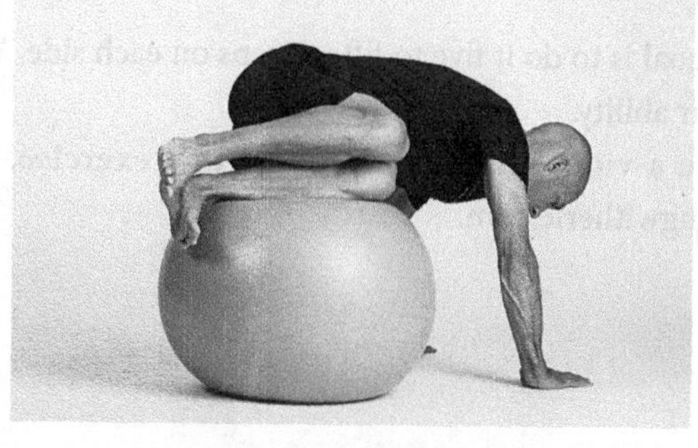

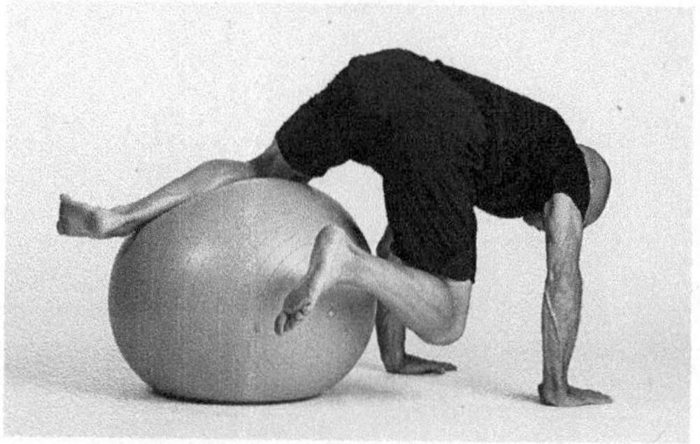

To perform, start with legs bent at ninety degrees, left one on the Fitball, right stacked above, and your arms shoulder width apart on the floor. From this starting position, roll the ball to the left by pressing your left knee into it, while your right leg drops off to the side of the ball near the floor. Return to start. Repeat. Do all your reps on one side before switching over to the other side.

- Keep knees at ninety degrees the entire time. This is key. Feel it and be aware of it.
- Support your body with the leg that is on the ball throughout the movement.
- Maintain a tight stomach.
- This is a total body strength exercise. Like the jackknife, this exercise engages everything, including a little more in the hips, and requires great body awareness and strength.

It's quite possible you won't be able to perform this one at first. It can be a future goal then, after you master knee toggle.

- Your goal is to do it five to fifteen reps on each side. Work to your ability.
- To see a video demonstration of this exercise, visit runningwitheric.com.

3. TOES TO CHEST (ADVANCED EXERCISE)

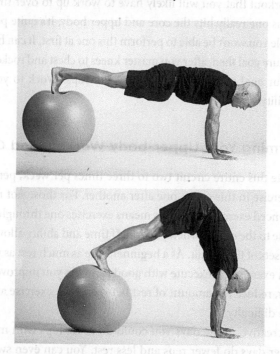

To perform, assume a plank position, placing your toes on top of the Fitball and your arms in a push-up position, elbows locked. Now pull your toes (and the ball) toward your arms while keeping your legs straight. Your glutes will rise up toward the ceiling and your body will become an inverted V. Hold that position for one to two seconds; then return to the start.

- Be sure you keep your toes on the top of the center of the ball.
- When you're at the top of the V, keep your elbows straight.
- Your legs have to be straight the whole time, especially at the height of your movement. If your back sags, you're not ready for this.
- Move in a controlled and fairly slow way, but work up to an increasing range of motion. The stronger you get, the more you should bring your body weight over your arms and shoulders.

- Like the two other advanced exercises, this is a whole-body workout that you will likely have to work up to over time. This one really hits the core and upper body. It's quite possible you won't be able to perform this one at first. It can be a future goal then, after you master knees to chest and rockers.
- Your goal is to do it eight to twenty reps. Work to your ability.

Performing Your Upper-body Workout and Circuit

Complete this entire circuit two to three times per week, performing each exercise in this order, one after another. For those not ready for the advanced exercises (*)—this means exercises one through seven—add these to the circuit when you can. If time and ability allow, do two to three sets of the circuit. As a beginner, take as much rest as you need between exercises to execute with good form. As you improve and get stronger, reduce the amount of rest between each exercise and set to increase difficulty.

Get creative. Some days you could do more reps with more rest, and other days do fewer reps and less rest. You can even switch this up from set to set. When you are short on time, pick two to three of these exercises and perform them to fatigue. You can achieve a lot in ten to fifteen minutes.

1. Knees to chest
2. Windshield wipers
3. Scorpions
4. Iso bridge
5. Knee toggle
6. Frog crunch
7. Rockers
8. Jackknife (*)
9. Can opener (*)
10. Toes to chest (*)

Sequencing Foot/Leg Strength and Upper-body Workouts

Should I work foot and leg muscles the same day as upper body? Do I do them individually? How do I integrate strength training with my runs? Can I run and strength-train the same day? These are some of the questions I hear most frequently, so I'm sure you're wondering about it all just about now. There's no right answer or perfect schedule, but I'll highlight for you the preferred sequencing over a week, knowing there will be some days you have easy, light-intensity runs, and other days when you're really pushing yourself hard out there on the run.

Okay, so it's best to perform your foot/leg strength circuits on days when you also have your more intense runs—and preferably do these circuits immediately after your run. At first blush, this may seem counterintuitive, but think about it: If you do both the same day, you allow your feet and legs (and glutes) to recover on the off days. In contrast, if you do a high-intensity run one day, a foot/leg circuit the next, high-intensity run the third, and on and on, your muscles never get a shot to recover.

Now, your upper-body circuit training optimally will be performed on easy run days, whether before or after your run, it makes little difference. By following this sequencing, you're basically alternating days of lower- and upper-body strength training. On occasion, once a week, you can do it all together (but on an easy run day).

Here's a sample weekly schedule of how to sequence and space your workouts. It's matched to the run schedule that follows later. Again, I am scheduling these by circuits, so remember to do them when you have time, but when you don't, pick a few of the exercises to perform that day. Some of you may have more time during the week than on weekends, or vice versa. Shuffle the days to match your time availability.

Day 1: one to three upper-body circuits
Day 2: foot/leg/glute circuit

Day 3: one to three upper-body circuits

Day 4: foot/leg/glute circuit

Day 5: no-strength-training day

Day 6: upper-body and/or foot/leg/glute (combo)

Day 7: no-strength-training day

This is not an ironclad schedule. A lot of what you'll do requires your own self-guidance. And remember, have fun.

4

PERFORMANCE RUNNING

THE NEXT MORNING, we meet at Jackson Hole High School, specifically the track/football stadium. Go, Broncs! I see you rolling those shoulders, the occasional hitch in your step. After some strength training, it's natural to feel muscles in places you didn't even know you had muscles. Remember, you get it where you need it.

Why does that track entrance gate snake back and forth? you ask. Got to keep all that big, four-legged wildlife from stomping up the grounds. To a moose, the pleasant, always green artificial turf looks like a field of heaven. For us, it's perfect to begin working on your form with some barefoot running.

Not to be cute, but I describe the ideal of the running form you'll soon be learning as "performance" because "form" is at the heart of the word. Without form, there's no performance, full stop.

Some runners argue that they don't need to work on form. They have all kinds of reasons: "I'm not serious enough to need to learn"; "Nobody taught me how to run in the first place"; "I've been running fine for years"; "My body runs as it should." I understand. But why not challenge yourself? See how good it can feel to reinvent your run form. Also, if you've been suffering from aches and pains and even injuries associated with your running, there's a reason, and one of the root causes is likely poor form.

Our bodies are designed to move in a certain way, common to all of us, and because of this I fundamentally believe there is a single "best" form for running. Yes, some may have more innate ability to run than others (just like in other sports). But with the proper instruction in form, you can learn to run to the best of your ability, with the greatest efficiency.

Think of sprinters. They spend years honing their form and technique, focusing on the slightest movements to improve their time by hundredths of a second. If you watch the Olympics or any other track-and-field event featuring the hundred-meter dash, you'll see that all of these sprinters look the same when racing, from the moment they start, to picking up speed, to the final burst down the stretch. They have the same form, because it's clear to any in the sport what the most efficient way to sprint is. And sprinting is running.

But then go to a marathon. Ignore the elite runners in the front of the pack, and watch everybody else. They move every which way. No other sport works like this. Tennis, golf, and swimming—all these activities teach form as fundamental to training. Why? Because the right technique translates into performance gains.

Running is no different, and there are biomechanical studies that detail the efficiencies of proper foot strike, arm carriage, and the like. More than trying to improve performance, though, I believe running with good form is important because it trains your body into its natural state of equilibrium, allowing you to layer on the advantages of strength training. Important as well—particularly to those who struggle with tightness, aches, and pains—form will lead you down a path where you're running at ease. Sounds spectacular, I know.

Now, here's the good news: Learning proper run form is easy. There are five stages to the run stride: foot strike, leg stance, knee drive, takeoff, and arm carry. Once you learn these, you have the knowledge you need.

Here's the bad news: Executing good run form consistently is hard work. Mastery is not won through more knowledge, but rather through constant awareness and practice that you are running the best you can with proper form.

At first, you have to be aware of each of the five parts of every stride. You'll likely be tense. That's to be expected. Over time and through infinite practice (I still work at it in every run), your thinking about good form becomes subconscious. You're still aware, but it's at a level of feeling. If your form is right or wrong, you'll feel it. I used to train triathletes in swim form, and every experienced swimmer I met at the pool would tell me the same thing: They could simply feel a bad stroke and adjust accordingly. Running is no different.

What is this feeling? Muscle memory. Your body learns what is right and wrong with such mastery that your conscious mind no longer plays much of a part. Do you think about walking or riding a bike or writing? No, of course not. Yet think of the orchestration of muscles required to do these activities. This is muscle memory in action. The beautiful thing is that through awareness and practice, you can retrain your muscles, reformat that memory, to do what you want.

Learning good form in and of itself is not the challenge ahead of you. Instead the ultimate goal is realizing this muscle memory. And there is no end point, no complete mastery; once you achieve proper form, you just keep practicing it. But apply the basics first. You'll straightaway realize gains in the efficiency of your stride, then improve, improve, improve. I look at good form as something to be perfected and enjoyed over a lifetime.

Since we're focusing on form today, I bet you're wondering why I brought the slant board and a pair of ski poles to the track. We covered strength training, you might say. But you'll see why I brought them in a minute. Take off those shoes and socks again and hop onto the board with your left foot. We'll start with some stability exercises. You can't remove strength from form. One helps the other, same as the strategic running foundation to come next. Not only will the slant board give you the ability to maintain proper form, but it also aids in developing that precious muscle memory.

As you work the slant board, know one thing: All of us, regardless of our running ability or experience, can benefit from reshaping or fine-tuning our form. As you run—and afterward—your body will feel better. That's a performance gain every type of runner can appreciate, and something, unfortunately, the laboratory can't prove.

Once you start feeling those muscles warm up, let's move over to the turf. I want to watch you closely, examine your form, and see where you can improve. Soon, though, you'll need to focus on it yourself. It is your own awareness of how you run—and should run—that will make the difference.

COMMON RUN FORM MISTAKES

Take it nice and slow around the inside of the track. Feel your body; be aware of your movements: where your bare foot strikes the turf first. Pay attention to the length of your stride, the way you carry your upper body, the lift of your knees, your push off the ground with your foot. Then just let go of all of this and sense how your form feels—natural or not?

Come on back. Take a seat. You'll be working those legs plenty today. No need for me to break down exactly what you're doing wrong. I want you to ask yourself that question. But know this: If your stride feels natural to you, it doesn't necessarily mean you have proper form. In fact, once we transform how you run, it will probably feel unnatural at first. You'll be fighting muscle memory that has become entrenched with your run form mistakes.

There are all kinds of improper form. See if any of the most common ones listed below (and the issues they cause) match your own. Further, go out and watch other runners; detect the good and bad with their technique. It's helpful insight into your own form and works to heighten your awareness.

- *Heel strikers*—Runners who land on their heels first. This creates instability, placing a lot of emphasis on the quad muscles. It causes a slow cadence and doesn't allow for the athletic engagement of the feet, which then keeps the calves from firing appropriately. All of this leads to IT band issues, tight hip flexors, and a weak gluteus medius.

- *Overstriders*—Runners who strike their lead foot too far out in front of their bodies. Often they are heel strikers as well. That said, you can still overstride when striking flat footed or forefooted. The foot still extends past the knee when striking the ground, and these runners land with pointed toes or on the outside of their foot. They typically suffer from a slow cadence and instability at the knee/hip/glute.
- *Benders*—Runners who keep their knees too bent throughout their gait (very common among barefoot runners and runners who do not pick up the pace very often). By not straightening the legs over the course of their stride, benders overstress the quads, forcing their dominance, while disengaging activation of the gluteus medius and calves. Benders often find they have knee pain, IT band pain, and very tight hip flexors.
- *Swingers*—Runners who swing their leg to the side and out, making little half circles with each stride, rather than lifting the leg. There's a lot of hip movement, but with an absence of knee drive, they suffer many of the same issues as benders and heel strikers.
- *Leaners*—Runners who bend forward from the waist or lean too far forward with their upper body. This typically forces the knees to remain bent throughout the stride, limiting core and glute engagement, thereby losing structural foundation.
- *Bouncers*—Runners who bounce up and down with each stride rather than looking to keep their shoulders level. This creates a disproportionate amount of knee drive and/or force into the ground compared to one's speed (i.e., power is expended moving up and down instead of propelling forward). In a word, it is inefficient.

- *High kickers*—Runners who kick too high behind their body or push off backward (akin to pawing the ground with the foot). This negates knee lift/drive, and can cause leaning issues.

Where does this improper form come from? Everybody is different. Essentially, our running is a product of our past experience. Shoes with built-up heels play a big role, but we'll get into that later. Understand, though, I know plenty of barefoot runners with bad form, so there is no magic bullet in just stripping off those shoes. Your athletic or training background influences form. You may have built up some muscles over others, and this shaped how you run.

Don't focus on the source of your mistakes. Commit to understanding and having the patience to correct them by executing proper form. And trust me: I know what this takes. When I came out to Denver and started doing some long runs, I never questioned my form. Then one day, coming back into town, I ran past some storefront windows. I couldn't believe the reflection staring back at me. This runner looked awful. There was no smoothness in his movements, only an awkward lumbering on his heels. Was this me? I asked myself. I imagined myself still running like I had during my gridiron days, gliding across the field, fluid, at ease, or sprinting down the backstretch of the track during a 4 X 100 relay.

Back home, I went through some old football tapes. I wasn't crazy. When I had the ball, sprinting down the field, there was that smoothness. But whenever I came back to the huddle or to the sideline, there was that lumbering runner again. So I began to examine my form as a sprinter and attempted to mimic this, just at a slower speed. I eliminated my heel strike, drove higher with my knees, and then got my leg down straight. Day after day, month after month, I trained and practiced, refining my form, developing muscle memory so that I could return to what I knew athletic running, performance running, to be.

Here's what I want you to do before we go into the elements of proper run form: Go out in your regular shoes and have someone take some quick snapshots of you from the side as you run. Photos are better than video, because you'll see in stop-motion the exact position of your feet, legs, hips, upper body, and head throughout your stride. Then compare this to the proper run form photos that you'll soon see in this book. (You can use the photos you take again later to compare to shots you take of yourself after you're into the drills and program to reshape your form. They'll help you see the changes you make as you learn proper form.)

Now, despite my breakdown of common run form mistakes, I want to make one more point clear: The remedies for these are not individual in the making. In my opinion, I think we tend to overcomplicate things by thinking that every mistake or running issue has a unique drill or solution. I get it. Most of us think we have "special" issues or a singular type of injury. But I have to tell you that I have conducted more than a thousand training sessions with runners, and most have the same issues, no matter their cause (shoe or otherwise), and they all tend to lead back to muscle disequilibrium and improper form. Therefore, most different running problems have the same remedy, which is achieved through strength and form work.

There's comfort in this, I believe. In a very real way, we're all in this together. By following a common practice, we can all improve; we can all do better.

PROPER RUN FORM

Now, I'm going to let you in on a secret: I brought you here for the soft turf, but also to show you pure athleticism and form in motion. Not from me. There's the whistle. Here they come: the grade-schoolers out here for gym class.

Children. Yes. Watch them run. Really be aware of their movements as they dash down the track, because they are illustrating what I want to teach you. Look how playful they are as they run: hopping, skipping, and laughing in between. True enjoyment. Also, look what else they're doing out here: jumping—often in pure glee. My young daughter is the same. From the time she was two years old, she was always running, always jumping—this is pure athleticism.

Guess what: The two are the same. Running is jumping, and we should do them the same way. When you jump, you drive your feet into the ground to go in the opposite direction. Same as running. The only difference is that in jumping we propel ourselves upward instead of forward. In both, we have two feet in the air at the same time.

Stand up. I want to further my point. Now jump in place. Again, try to go higher. One more time as high as you can, and be aware of what your body is doing. Okay, evaluate. When jumping, do we generate power and take off on our heels? No. Do we land on our heels? No. Do we land with our feet under our knees? Yes. When preparing to jump, you bend your knees to gain power, right? Yes. Are your knees in front of your body or behind it? In front.

Good, these answers are the beginning to understanding performance running. Pun intended, let's "jump" into the five stages of proper form. Concentrate on them one at a time. Taken together, these five stages are everything you need to know about proper run form.

Now, stride down the field, focusing only on striking the turf with your forefoot. . . .

1. Forefoot Strike

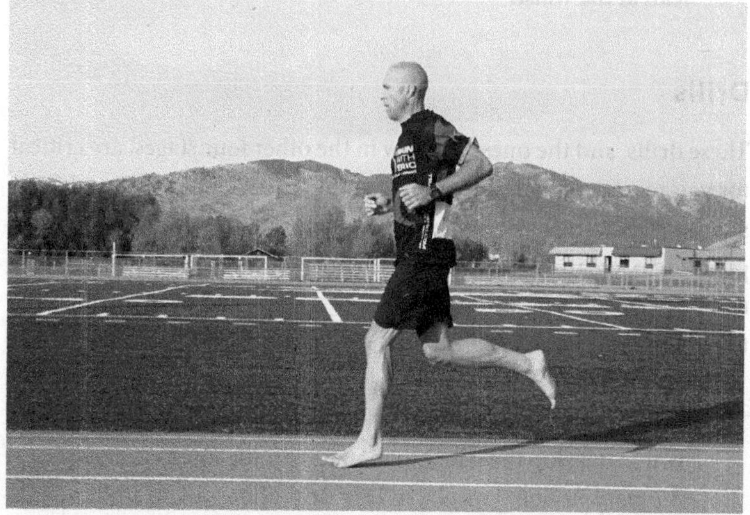

As in strength training, everything in proper form begins with the foot, specifically the forefoot. Landing there, as you see in the photograph, is the first line of stability in your stride. The toes, especially the big toe, engage the ground. The arch then fires, and you are creating a stable base that brings the knees and hips into alignment. By landing on the forefoot, your ankle, which should not extend past the knee, provides some shock absorption as your heel follows down. Striking with the forefoot also helps prevent you from overstriding (though it's no guarantee) and allows for a quicker cadence. When you work on form with bare feet, you really get a feel for all of this.

Technique and Awareness

- Strike the ground first with your forefoot.
- Keep your ankle under your knee. Don't ever let your foot reach so far out in front that your ankle is in front of your knee.
- Regardless of speed, the forefoot's strike in relationship to your body should not change.

- Your shoulders should stay in line with your hips; don't lean at the waist.

Drills

These drills, and the ones to follow in the other four stages, are critical for you to understand proper form and to experience how good form should "feel." They also serve to help you practice and reemphasize good form, creating the right muscle memory. As you progress, they can be performed as a warm-up before a run—and even during runs to get the right feel back.

- *Slant board/stability disk exercises*: The exercises will enable you to develop the strength to maintain the forefoot strike.
- *Barefoot jumping in place*: This drill allows us to understand and feel the foot strike from the forefoot. Runners should strike first with the forefoot and then allow the heel to hit. The faster we run, and the stronger our feet become over time, the more the heel can stay elevated off the ground. But when first working on form, and when running slowly, you should allow the heel to drop to the ground after the forefoot.
- *Barefoot running in place*: You really can't run wrong while running in place. Without coaching or instruction, you'll do it well, especially when running in place fairly fast. We will naturally strike the ground with our forefoot, bring our knees out in front of us, and drive power directly into the ground. When running for real, the only thing that changes is that we angle our leg to the ground to propel us forward, rather than up and down in place. This is also a perfect drill to understand how we should drive through the ground and lift our knees in front of us.

2. Leg Stance

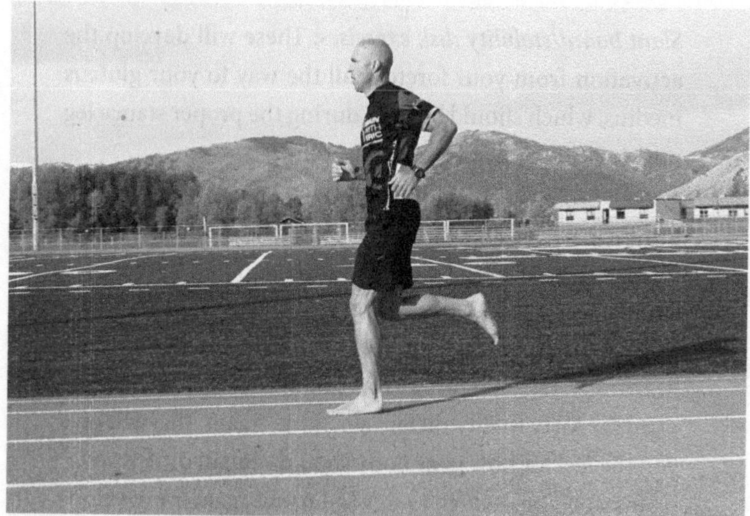

Although the transition from forefoot strike to knee drive (stage three) takes only a split second, it is essential to execute proper form when you do it. Notice how the stance leg (my left in the photo) supports your whole body, which should remain upright, with no lean at the waist. This prevents stress on the ankle and calf and allows for a quick turnover to the knee drive. With this leg stance position, the muscle activation begun with the forefoot strike now continues up the calf. The knee, and especially the gluteus medius, is stabilized, and the whole body is supported, fostering muscle equilibrium and efficiency.

Technique and Awareness

- After your forefoot strike, allow your heel to touch the ground.
- Feel the stabilization from your feet to your knees, hips, and glutes.
- The stance leg remains almost directly under the body.
- The body remains upright, with no lean or bending at the waist.

Drills

- *Slant board/stability disk exercises*: These will develop the activation from your forefoot all the way to your gluteus medius, which should be fired during the proper stance leg position to stabilize your lower body.
- *Barefoot strides*: By training barefoot, you'll get the proper feel for your heel dropping after your forefoot strike. Perform five to ten strides at a moderate speed for ten to twenty seconds at a time on grass or artificial turf to get the feel for dropping your heel after your forefoot strike.
- *Marching*: Yes, marching. You can march in place or forward for forty to fifty meters at a time. Again, this will give you the feel for how your body should remain directly over your stance leg. Return to this again and again for developing the right muscle memory.

3. Knee Drive

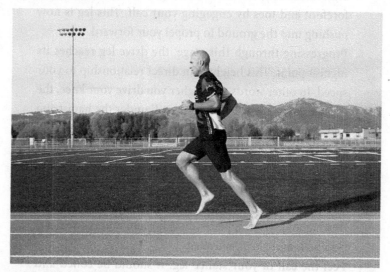

In the first two stages, forefoot strike and leg stance, you were focusing on the movement and placement of only one leg: the stance leg. Now you have to be aware of both as you push your stance leg into the ground, while lifting up your drive leg (my right in the photos). This stage promotes stabilization throughout the body while providing power to propel us forward.

Two key actions come into play here: One, your stance leg stabilizes and directs power into the ground relative to your speed. (The degree of angle represents how fast you are going.) Two, the calf muscle of your stance leg engages to prepare you to take off on your forefoot and toes again. The visualizations I provide after drills are key to getting the form right on this one.

TECHNIQUE AND AWARENESS

- On the drive leg, lift your knee forward and up. Keep your ankle relaxed and under the hamstring so that it is not reaching in front of you or past your knee. The knee leads the way.

- Simultaneously, on the stance leg, transition onto your forefoot and toes by engaging your calf. This leg is now pushing into the ground to propel your forward.
- Progressing through this stage, the drive leg reaches its highest point. This height is in direct relationship to your speed. In other words, the higher you drive your knee, the greater your speed. The ankle is still under the hamstring and behind the knee.
- At the same time, the stance leg almost straightens, and you are now on your toes, still pushing power into the ground (and not pushing off backward). Your hip is open, and you're not leaning over at the waist.
- Throughout, your upper body is upright and relaxed, abdominals and glutes activated.
- Feel the calf of your stance leg. It should be coiled and ready to provide power in the next stage.

Drills

- *Slant board/stability disk movement training*: The knee lift and run squat with rotation exercises are key to developing the strength and muscle memory you'll need to execute this stage of the running stride. Foot and calf strength are vital for this stage, used when you return to the forefoot to take off forward. All foot exercises help this.
- *Barefoot running in place (again)*: Watch how you drive your knee upward while at the same time transferring power into the ground through your stance leg.
- *Hurdles*: Run quickly over self-made hurdles of eight to twelve inches in height spaced approximately a foot apart. This will force you to drive the knee high and provide power into the ground with your stance leg.
- *Marching (again)*: Keep your knees high like a good soldier, and your legs straight for stability. Let your foot go up on

its toes as you march; do not stay flat-footed. Work that muscle memory.

- *Skipping for distance*: This will force you to drive your knee upward, and show you how the height of your knee correlates to power with the stance/takeoff leg.
- *Hill sprints*: Run uphill with hands held behind your neck. This will push you to raise your knees and to feel your core and glutes engage.

4. Takeoff

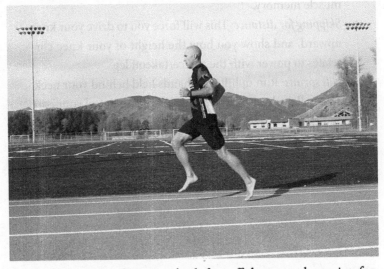

You are jumping in this stage, both feet off the ground, moving forward. Like a jump, you are using the energy coiled in your muscles from the prior stage. This energy, translated into speed, is dictated by the distance between your drive leg knee and stance leg foot (the higher the knee, the steeper the stance leg, the greater the power and the faster your speed). This is important to note, because in this stage you're also beginning the cycle again with the other leg (i.e., the drive leg), moving into position for the forefoot strike. You do not reach out with the drive leg to strike the ground farther away from you to gain speed in a longer stride. The forefoot strike placement should always be straight down and the same, regardless of speed.

Technique and Awareness

- With your stance leg foot, you need only push off slightly with your toes. The power comes from your stance leg's neutral ankle and calf engagement as you drive into the ground. Don't point your toes by pushing off with your ankle.

- Your drive leg rises to its high point (relative to speed), then transitions to an almost ninety-degree angle, your foot still slightly behind your knee and under your hamstring. Do not reach out too far with the foot before landing. Be patient; allow the ground to come to you to begin your forefoot strike.
- As your forefoot strikes the ground with the drive leg, it becomes the stance leg and stabilizes the body.
- Keep your posture tall and straight and your hips open.

Drills

- *Slant board/stability disk movement training*: As in the previous stage, the knee lift and run squat with rotation exercises will develop the strength and muscle memory you'll need to execute this stage of the running stride.
- *Skipping for distance*: On flat terrain, skip. Gradually, build the distance of your skips to your maximum range. This will give you the feeling of powering off into the air, while bringing your other leg down. Plus, it helps build leg strength.
- *Running stairs/hill sprints*: Dash up a flight of stairs or hill fast and powerfully, with high knees. Practice powerful takeoffs, extending your leg straight and driving power into the ground with each step. This exercise is fantastic at mimicking the entire run gait.

5. Arm Carry

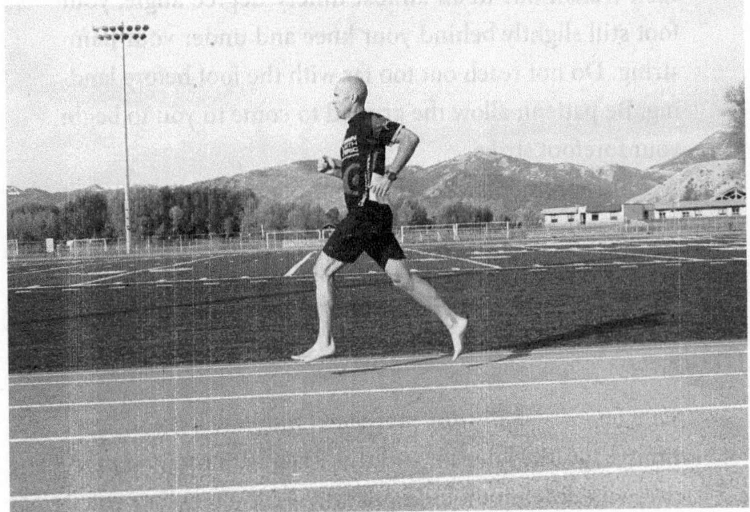

By swinging your arms forward and back through the run-stage cycles, you allow yourself to open up your chest and keep your shoulders square, increasing your efficiency, and easing your ability to breathe. Avoid letting your arms cross your body and turning your shoulders side to side. With proper carriage, you work your arms and legs in unison. This creates fluidity in your stride and a relaxed whole body. As you speed up, you can extend your arms for leverage and power, whether in a sprint or the last kick to the line.

Technique and Awareness

- Keep your arms bent at a ninety-degree angle.
- Drive your elbows back and keep them close to your torso.
- Do not swing your arms too far in front of you. Let there be a natural cadence that matches your legs' movement.
- Relax your upper body, arms, shoulders, and hands. A relaxed runner is a fast runner.
- Keep your arms swinging in one plane, forward and back, not across your body.

- Imagine running with dumbbells in your hands; intuit how your body naturally finds the most economical way to carry them. You would keep your elbows bent and arms short to lessen the strain as much as possible.

Those are the five stages to good form. Let them settle into your mind as you lace those shoes back on. We'll drive out of town down Highway 22 for a run along the Snake River. The path is a bit rocky, but it's as flat a terrain as you'll find out here in Jackson.

SUPPORT FOR PROPER RUN FORM

Visualizations

Seeing form in your mind's eye is a powerful technique in mastering good run form. These visualization techniques can be used as a drill during warm-ups, but can and should also be used whenever you're running to practice active awareness. Whenever you need to reinforce good form and to continue to develop muscle memory, use these visualizations.

- *Field of logs.* For proper knee drive, imagine yourself crossing a field of logs spaced evenly apart. With each running step, you drive the knee high to step over a log. The faster your speed, the larger the log, but keep that foot under your hamstring.
- *Cowboy and rope.* For proper upper-body posture, visualize that a Wyoming cowboy has a rope around your waist and you are pulling him along.
- *Bow and arrow.* In this run stage, it is important to be aware of both legs. As you are providing power through the ground, you are also thinking about driving the other knee forward. This is similar to the action of a bow and arrow. The cocked arm pulling the bowstring back is your knee

drive leg. The straight arm holding the bow rigid is your stance leg. Together, they provide the power and stabilization to propel you forward. Look up at the photo again and you can see this. Visualize this bow-and-arrow action of your legs as you run.

Cadence

Crucial to the execution of the five stages of run form is proper cadence. No matter your height, your foot should strike the ground roughly twenty-two to twenty-three times every fifteen seconds.

Runners commonly focus too much on their stance leg when trying to increase cadence. Trying to be quick, they slap the ground with their stance leg. The opposite should be done. Work on being quick with the knee drive leg to increase cadence. Think like Bruce Lee and his one-inch punch that could send men flying across the room. He said he developed this power not by how hard he hit someone, but rather with how quickly he pulled back his punch (just like the knee drive, but be sure the stance leg goes almost straight, not too bent; think bow and arrow).

Now, don't try to work on cadence while simultaneously focusing on each stage of run form. Sometimes too much is too much. Instead, during your easy runs, concentrate on your cadence every five to ten minutes. Do your counts and slow up/down accordingly. Over time, through practice, you will begin to feel proper cadence and will no longer need to count as much.

The Right Shoes and the Wrong Shoes

Look at that water. The Snake River flows pretty well this time of year. That's all cold, clear runoff from the mountains. Farther downstream, you'll get some good class-three rapids. While you're out here, definitely sign up for a white-water trip. It's a thrill to paddle into a swirl of thunderous river.

Okay, so I want to talk shoes, because they're the culprits for many of the running issues I encounter—or at least the development of them. I haven't made mention of yours yet, but now, well, I need to be frank. Maybe these are your old ones; they have some wear and tear. Maybe you've bought a new minimalist pair since, but you were worried about our trails out here eating them up. But it's time for you to realize that your shoes with the big heel, all that "stabilization"—they're breaking you down as a runner even as they likely advertise that they're helping you keep from breaking down.

As I've said, I'm not a barefoot-running purist who believes that you should run this way twenty-four/seven. Barefoot running has its purposes, particularly in the strength exercises and form practice we've done. Running barefoot is a great way to feel your toes, feet, and arches, to get a sense of how they need to engage in your stride. It's also a great way to build strength and endurance.

But I am a coach—one who helps runners perform well in races—and it's very hard to train and perform appropriately without adequate protection for your feet. The Tarahumara know to wear some kind of protection while traversing their terrain over many miles. So should we.

There's protection; then there's the kind of shoes that no doubt you and millions of others have bought, with the gargantuan heels and thick soles that try to cushion our feet and somehow give us proper stability. They're problematic for lots of reasons: They inhibit the natural movement of your foot; they don't allow you to engage your foot for stability or proper muscle activation; they weigh too much; and most of all, they elevate the heel. This last one is a disaster.

We're out on the trail with your big-heeled shoes. Try to forefoot strike. Not easy, right? You have to almost force yourself to do it, and even then, your calves aren't engaging completely because your heel hits the ground too soon. That means you're not getting the stability and muscle activation you need from your forefoot to your knees to the glutes. Equally bad, when you heel strike, the calves do not fire as they should, which translates into a loss of power, elasticity, and an overstressing of the quads.

Come to a stop. I want to show you the clearest example of why running with an elevated heel is a real problem. Jump up and down on your forefoot. Remember how springy you were at the track doing this barefoot? Not so much now in your high heels. Our calves act as loaded springs, storing and releasing energy as we jump or run. The calves need to be loaded (or what I call "on stretch") to release this energy, giving us a springy feeling. This can't take place in high-heeled shoes because the heel hits the ground too soon, not allowing the calves to remain on stretch—an energy zapper. And because of this, the knee can be thrown forward, giving us that quad dominance and poor glute recruitment. Now I hope you understand why runners need to transition away from shoes with elevated heels. Better form, more power, less injury.

The importance of our shoes in run form has made sense to me for a long time, but it never struck home more than when I watched my daughter. For the first four years of her life, the only shoe I could find for her was a flat, almost zero-drop shoe. By zero drop, I mean the sole has the same thickness from the heel to the toe box. Barefoot, or in these shoes, she ran beautifully: natural form all the way, forefoot and all. Then, when she was five years old, shoes with elevated heels were all over the place, and zero-drop ones were almost nonexistent for her. In fact, shoe manufacturers were pretty much promoting bad running form by rigging their thick-soled shoes with flashing cool lights that lit up only when the heel was struck. And when my daughter ran in these shoes, she became a heel striker. Terrible.

Is there a perfect shoe? I'm not sure, but I do know there are wrong shoes. And what shoe companies ironically call a "traditional" shoe (i.e., one with lots of stabilization, a thick sole, and a twelve- to fifteen-millimeter difference from heel to toe) is most definitely the wrong shoe. In the store they may feel comfortable, but watch out when you're running. And once you get those feet bomber strong, you will wonder how you ever ran in them in the first place.

Then there is what I like to call a "performance" shoe: zero drop, thin sole, and flexible. This kind of shoe allows for proper forefoot strike, awareness of form, stability through the toes and foot, and the lengthening of the calves to act as a spring. Further, by running in them, you foster foot strength and muscle equilibrium through the body, because you are able to use your feet better.

Look again at the Tarahumara. They run in old tire treads cut to the fit of their foot, nothing more securing them than a leather strap between their toes and around their ankle. In my own life, I've run in just about every kind of shoes of different make and design—elevated heels, minimal heel, zero drop, low profile, high profile, stability, no stability. Never have my feet been stronger, my stability better, or my body more attuned—and pain-free—than in a performance shoe as I've described it. When doing the majority of your running in zero-drop shoes and in concert with foot strength and form, you will start to notice a difference in muscle distribution in your hips and a significant reduction in hip flexor tightness.

But if you're still not sure, just try it. Run in the right shoe; experiment with a zero-drop performance shoe. Feel how much easier it is to maintain proper form, and how much stronger you become as a runner.

But don't just toss out your old shoes and start running every day in a zero-drop shoe. You have to take the transition slowly from a traditional shoe to a performance shoe, because you'll be firing muscles that aren't used to being fired. At first, use the zero-drop shoes for shorter runs, and your old ones for longer runs. Then gradually increase distance in the former. As your feet and calves become stronger, with exercises and better form, your old shoes will become more and more uncomfortable, and that is the sign that you can probably transition away from them completely. To ease the change, follow the performance running transition workouts that I'll detail for you later.

Right now, if you're wondering why I'm digging into my backpack, I have some good news. Because you've come out to Jackson to train with me, I've ordered you a pair just your size to get you started down the right path to the right shoe. I'd love for you to wear them today, so we can really work on form.

Here they are. . . . Cool, huh? But cool as they are, a final note: There's no ideal shoe for every situation. When road running, a zero-drop performance shoe like this one is likely all the protection you'll need. But if you're hitting the trail, they will probably not shield your feet enough. We need to be smart; rocks hurt. Just as barefoot running is not always appropriate, same with minimal shoes. So if you need a thicker sole because of the terrain, wear one, but try to choose one that is zero drop or as minimal as possible that still provides the protection you need. As long as you do most of your running in zero-drop shoes and always focus on good form, it's okay at times to sacrifice some flexibility to get the protection you need.

Okay, time to get cracking on training you for proper form.

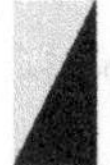

Paragons of Form—The Tarahumara Indians

If you watch the Tarahumara cross Copper Canyon, whether uphill, downhill, or over the riverbed, they're always maintaining proper form. They are picture-perfect in the truest sense of the term. Why? How?

Well, they start, even as kids, wearing their huaraches, which promote good foot strike and allow the calves to work across their full range of motion. They never get thrown off by all the high-tech, thick-soled, elevated-heel shoes with zippy logos that our children wear. And when they were tempted by sponsorship at the Leadville 100, they ditched the "traditional" shoes during the race for their performance huaraches.

Then there's terrain. Again, from their childhood onward, they are doing long, sustained hill climbs in Copper Canyon. Hello, foot and leg strength and muscle memory. On these climbs, they're basically doing the natural version of slant board exercises, especially the knee drives, while perfecting their form.

The Tarahumara also have their now famous ball game, rarajípari. More specifics on this in our next training session, but the game promotes lots of sprinting, which is great for fostering proper toeing off, as well as hip and leg extension. Further, they play rarajípari on very uneven, grassy fields pocked with stones and divots that demand the quick lifting of their feet and knees. No smooth, obstacle-free terrain for them, allowing for the shuffling of feet or swinging legs. They learn proper form as kids or they're constantly tripping and falling.

TRAIN FOR FORM

Now, before we head down the path to start cracking on good run form, go back over what I showed you at the track. I want you to close your eyes and see yourself running with proper form. Really see it, like you're an observer alongside the river, watching the two of us run past. Visualize yourself through each of the five stages of proper form. See yourself executing each stage properly and with ease.

All right, do you have it?

Come on, then. Give it a try, all together now: forefoot strike, leg stance, knee drive, takeoff. And again, always with the arm carry, back and forth. Keep focusing; be aware of how your body is moving.

Nice job, but remember to drive those knees. Even though you know everything you need to about good form, this won't be easy. Remember: Be patient. If you've been running one way for a long time, it takes some effort to learn another way so that it eventually feels natural.

I won't be here to tell you whether you're doing everything right or wrong. That's okay. I don't need to be. Even with athletes I train in person or remotely around the world, I'm constantly repeating myself, saying the same things that I told you in the breakdown of the five stages. You know what to do. Repetition, repetition, repetition is the only way to get it right.

Understand the stages individually, see yourself doing them, and then execute again and again. Get the feeling and do it over and over, telling yourself throughout: foot strike, leg stance, knee drive, take-off, arm carry. It will come. As with strength training, take to form training like a martial artist. Small steps and awareness will get you there. And as I recommended before, keep taking photos of yourself to evaluate your progress.

How you make the transition to performance running depends on many things, including your present form and foot and leg strength. If you're a longtime heel striker, you'll experience some calf soreness, and the forefoot strike will feel awkward. Just as strength training creates muscle equilibrium, so too does performance running. The form I've taught you is how your body is meant to move. Over time, your body will feel better, less tight, less fatigued. Proper form takes away all those common running aches and pains, and will enhance your speed and overall performance. Trust the coaching; it's worth the effort.

To get the form right when you take it out for a spin day after day, start by doing the performance running transition workouts that follow. They will ease and speed your transition to proper form. Second, throughout the transition and beyond, do your strength-training program. Third, whenever you feel like you need to reinforce good run form mechanics, do the drills I have listed in each of the five stages of run form. Together, they will develop for you the muscle memory and equilibrium that make proper form not only possible, but enduring for your lifetime as a runner. Everything works together in this program to support natural running.

Performance Running Transition Program

The following schedule and drills will aid you through your change in shoes and reshaping your run form. It's best to make this transition when you can be patient and don't feel the demand to put in a lot of miles. If you're gearing up for some races, it's probably not the best time to begin. Instead, try to use this program at the start of a season, when your mileage is reduced. Finally, if you've just come off a long season of running, your body needs to rejuvenate. Take a couple weeks off, no running at all, before launching into this program.

1. Schedule

The goal is four runs per week at a length of thirty minutes. Begin with a five-to-ten-minute run to see how your body responds to the new form, and build from there. These should be light, easy runs where the focus is on form, cadence, and a low heart rate. If you're not able to breathe only through your nose, you're pushing it too hard. And, since you're taking it slow, wear your new performance shoes. Once you are comfortable for ten minutes, add five minutes every week or so to build up to a half hour. This program should take roughly four to six weeks.

2. Awareness Drills

While building to your thirty minutes, do the drills highlighted in each of the five stages of run form to help you understand how your body should move, and to develop good run form muscle memory. Work on them when time allows (not as a day-to-day routine), whether as a warm-up or part of your runs. For those of you just beginning, take it very slowly with these drills. As with the distance of your runs, you need to work up to sprints and quick hill climbs.

A couple final notes of advice on your run form transition and overall training. First, a word of caution for those who use treadmills. I know, believe me: Sometimes you just have to hit the treadmill at home or in the local gym, particularly during those frigid winter months or wet days, to keep to your schedules. I get it, and I actually like the treadmill in the winter for speed training. But you should know that maintaining good form on a treadmill is very difficult, especially the knee drive stage. Extra attention, extra awareness must be focused on driving the knee forward and up immediately after the foot strike, because the moving track will want to take your stance leg back before you toe off. To be clear, I'm not saying don't run on a treadmill. I'm saying that, if you do, pay attention to your knee drive, knee drive, knee drive—step over those logs.

Second, I have you running some hills, and unless you live on long stretches of flatland, you should. They're good for strength and helping with your form. But a lot of runners simply don't know what to do when running hills. They change form, they heel strike, and they do all kinds of funky things. Uphill or downhill, you should maintain proper form; nothing changes other than the grade.

This is easier uphill than downhill. When going uphill, be sure to focus on knee drive and not get lazy with it. Drive it uphill and feel that stance leg provide power into the ground. As your foot strength gets better, be sure to not let the heel drop too far to the ground; keep those calves fired, but with a quick cadence.

On downhill slopes, really focus on foot strike and not overstriding. At first you are going to have to slow down to achieve this. Run as slowly as you need to in order to maintain a good forefoot strike. In time you will get better and better, and your speed will improve along with your form. I find it helps to imagine myself pedaling a bike downhill. This helps get the knee drive, especially on steeper bits. Like everything else, the more you do it, the better you'll get at it.

Awareness and Form

You're doing great. Another short stretch. We don't want to push it too far the first day. Flow like the Snake River. Embrace that good form: foot strike, leg stance, knee drive, takeoff, arm carry.

Never put a time limit on success. You've already taken off down the path to proper form. Success and gains start immediately and continue infinitely—you just get better and better. It is not a light switch; it is a dimmer switch—you just keep getting the light brighter and brighter.

Okay, time to quiet and slow. Come to a walk. Look up there in the trees to your right. There, high up on a branch. A bald eagle. Majestic, right? And big. He's calm and focused up there, watching us, watching everything that passes, looking for lunch, perhaps.

Awareness. The eagle reminds us of that now. Awareness is everything when it comes to form. Feel your body; know what it is doing, how far you're striding, where your foot is striking, how you're carrying your arms, the straightness of your stance leg, the stability that comes from your big toe. All of it, whenever you run. The more you're aware of your form, the better you'll run. Through practice, this awareness of your form will become so natural to you that you'll be aware without being aware of it. Cool, right? Be like the bald eagle, watching always, calm, focused.

5

STRATEGIC RUNNING FOUNDATION

WE NEED MORE than endurance to run well for long distances; we need to be strong and fast. To build that, you need a well-rounded training schedule.

There will be a lot of words that follow about my strategic running foundation, but if you remember—and are convinced of—nothing else other than this philosophy, you're far ahead of many runners.

In the early afternoon of our fourth day together, we head out of Jackson, past Blacktail Butte. How are those calves feeling? If you've never had a forefoot strike, those few miles along the Snake River the day before will leave those legs with a little tenderness. That soreness is a sure sign you're on the way to a new, better form.

Look to the northeast. See anything in the shape of that ridgeline in the Gros Ventre Range? Still nothing? That's Sheep Mountain, but we locals call it the "Sleeping Indian." Ahh, see it now? That sharp angle on the ridge is the nose, the gentle slope downward his forehead, and that rounded bit at the center, his hands crossed across his chest. I know, cool. We cross into Grand Teton National Park, past a herd of elk—and the bigger herd of park visitors snapping pictures with their huge cameras (yes, they're big enough to be telescopes, and you're never quite sure whether it is Nat Geo or some guy from Georgia).

We turn down a gravel road toward Phelps Lake. You're lucky: Until a short while ago, nobody but members and guests of the Rockefeller family were allowed on this land, which the founder of Standard Oil bought for a song after the 1929 crash. Over the years, the family had donated most of the thirty-three thousand acres to the government. This was the last parcel they let go, and not far from here used to stand the Rockefeller lodge and cabins. Not a bad vacation spot.

Okay, let's do an easy warm-up run to Phelps Lake at the foot of Death Canyon. Enough history—we should talk about the future: your running future. You've worked—and will continue to—on foot strength, muscle equilibrium, and proper form. Now we'll put these to use. No matter what kind of runner you are—newbie to elite—you need to have a strong training foundation with which to realize your goals, and, let's face it, to run healthily. This means a system, a schedule of runs, strategically tailored to where you are at this moment to develop your endurance, strength, and speed together.

I coach runners of all abilities and distances throughout the world. So many of them came to me having never before followed a structured training plan. Once they bought into mine and trusted its purpose, they couldn't believe how nice it was to have all the guesswork taken off their hands, allowing them to focus on the day-to-day process. They embraced the schedule and became intoxicated by the structure and diversity it brought to their workouts.

You—just like they have—will likely derive a tremendous amount of satisfaction from the completion of each day's workout. And you will feel a similar satisfaction on finishing (or winning) a race, whether it's a 5K or an ultra, knowing the training got you there in the first place.

Just like strength and form, we can all benefit by building a solid training foundation. I'm talking everybody, at all levels. The elite unable to improve his race times. The veteran stuck doing the same thing all the time. The marathoner, never having worked speed or strength. The 10K'er lacking good kick at the end. Or the recreational runner finding his recreation not very recreational anymore. There's a tongue twister.

Now, Chris McDougall is a perfect example of the transformational power of the foundation work. After Chris and I bet in Denver that he could run with the Tarahumara and finish Copper Canyon, yes, we worked on his strength and form, but it was his strategic training that pulled everything together.

As I've said, Chris was a bit of a train wreck as a runner when we first met. Every stride was basically breaking him down. It was uncomfortable for him to run slowly, because of both his form and his inefficiencies at burning fat, so he would naturally speed up, because it felt better. Yet he could not maintain a fast pace because of a lack of strength, particularly his neuromuscular strength.

In short order, I had to prepare him for a fifty-mile race over tough, steep terrain. That meant he needed to build strength and running economy, while also developing his endurance abilities. If I had merely given him a schedule to up his miles every week, he would never have been able to do Copper Canyon. He needed a strength base on which to do those long miles.

For eight weeks, I put him through a regimen of short hill runs and sprints, fostering his strength while gradually increasing his miles. In two months, he was able to run almost ten hours a week, with his long run reaching almost four hours. On a cardiovascular level, he turned out to be more than capable, as most of us are. The key was giving his body the strength to handle those miles. That's where the strategy came into play. As he was injured all the time, it may seem counterintuitive to give him a series of hill runs and sprints, but it worked (and, given time constraints, it was the only thing to do).

After these first weeks, we concentrated on intervals and long, slow, sustained runs monitored by heart rate to economize his fat burning. Chris grew more confident in his running and more aware of how far, how hard he could push himself. Then, in the final eight weeks, we ramped up his speed endurance training, enabling him to run faster, longer, maximizing his engine to help the race pace feel easier, and his muscular endurance and efficiency to handle the terrain for fifty miles.

He crossed that finish line in Copper Canyon, and he achieved his bigger goal of building a lifelong running foundation to be able to do any type of run, long or short, fast or slow, on any given day.

Now, as you can tell when I talk about Chris, I'm a coach geek. I live and breathe this stuff. It's my passion to bring about leaps and bounds in performance, not just incremental improvement. So there's no reason that what constitutes a well-trained runner shouldn't be as plain to you as it is for me. And anyway, I wasn't always so clearheaded on this. Only when I started training triathletes in the Colorado winter did I realize the true benefit of offering my athletes more than a traditional endurance foundation base. Because of the cold and snowy weather in the early season, I couldn't ask my triathletes to keep putting in the miles outside, whether biking or running. During base building, I had to focus on higher-quality, greater speed/strength workouts that could be done inside or for shorter periods of time outside. These triathletes began performing better than they had when I gave them longer, higher-volume workouts. The experience made me realize that muscular strength and speed dictate endurance foundation and performance, not so much the other way around. Ever since, I've been working to develop the right mix of strength, raw speed, and endurance for their training foundation.

And a mix it is. Strength, speed, and endurance aren't separate entities. They complement one another, work and grow solid together, much like water, sand, and cement do in the creation of concrete.

I say "much like" because this analogy goes only so far, and I can already see some coaches, trainers, doctors, performance physiologists, and a slew of PhDs pulling at their hair, questioning my use of the terms strength, endurance, and speed. And they're right. There're so many layers and intersections with each of these words, and what I'll tell you to follow, that there's no way to explain the reasoning behind my methods with 100 percent completeness and accuracy without burying you in the science.

The good thing is, I'm here as your coach, not as a lecturer. I'm here to help you understand what kind of training regimen you should follow and why, not to prepare you for the medical boards. If I already have your faith, by all means, skip ahead to the training program itself. Many of my athletes do; then again, I understand the idea that knowledge is power.

In case you get lost, remember: We need more than endurance to run well for long distances; we need to be strong and fast.

THE FOUNDATION MIX

After a good two-mile run from my truck, we reach Phelps Lake. Yep, that's it: the clear blue jewel that appears amid the fir trees. Those Rockefellers, they knew how to live. Now this stretch of water is as much yours as theirs.

Okay, there's a level trail that runs right around the lake. I want you to go slowly, an easy pace, and I'll tell you about that mix.

Endurance

Your ability to go for as long as you need to go without breaking down—that's a pretty good definition of endurance. Now, this breakdown, it can happen in many ways: form, muscle, cardiovascular, fuel efficiency—which is where things begin to get complicated. We will train for the speed/strength endurance that will forestall breakdown.

Let's focus on what I mean by training for endurance alone. The most obvious part of this consists of cardiovascular conditioning. Many runners, perhaps after taking their twenties, even thirties off from hitting the road, find gaining this endurance tough going. In their first weeks, they're breathing heavily; their hearts are racing. This may seem the biggest hurdle to clear in training. And yes, it's critical, but the truth is that the cardio comes easiest for most runners. Put in some miles on a consistent basis and your breathing will ease; your heart will steady. It's very rarely the limiter on performance. To that point, have you ever heard of an ultramarathoner quitting a race because he was out of breath?

The other part of endurance alone centers on training your body to burn fat efficiently. I'm not talking so you'll lose weight. Sorry. Fat packs a lot of energy (more than carbs per calorie), and most of our bodies have enough of it to run several marathons in a row. But because of inefficiencies in burning it, our bodies can look to carbohydrates too much (or too soon) for fuel. This is a problem, because our stores of carbs are limited. If you become more efficient at burning fat, you'll run longer and have more endurance. This efficiency is realized by multiplying the number of mitochondria (little fat burners that produce energy) in your body. And that's the simple explanation.

Is there some multivitamin for increasing those mitochondria, becoming more efficient for greater endurance? Not so easy. But not so hard either.

By the way, when I told you to go at a slow pace around Phelps Lake, I didn't mean a moderate one. Ease it down a bit. A great many people don't know what it is to run slowly—and how necessary it is. For many it is uncomfortable to run slowly, so they just don't do it. Yes, uncomfortable, meaning it just doesn't feel right and you can't do it for long, often because of bad form and poor run economy.

Now, mitochondria love that slow pace; it's the perfect environment for them to multiply in. So, if you train slower, you become a more efficient fat burner, and you will be able to run longer, faster, using a more efficient fuel source. This gives you endurance. And to further help, your slow runs focused on fat burning give you the opportunity to work on developing good form, which enhances your efficiency as well. That's a nice loop.

Strength

We've already started on developing strength and muscle equilibrium. Through our strategic foundation, we focus on helping our muscles work better, more efficiently, to condition them for the endurance demands we'll put on them. This will allow you to run stronger, longer, at a higher level of effort.

That ultramarathoner I spoke about earlier: Why does he fail to finish? If it's not cardiovascular weakness, then what? Usually it's a lack of strength and economy. His muscles simply won't allow him to continue—or they're not able to handle a fast enough pace long enough to finish. Injury, fatigue, a lack of improvement—do not look for the culprit in your system's ability to pump oxygen throughout your body. Instead, look to muscular weakness and inefficiency.

In our strategic training, I concentrate on two kinds of strength, both critical to your improvement. The first is the obvious one: musculoskeletal strength. Our form training and work with the slant board, stability disks, and Fitball have already put us on the right path here. Like I've said, everything is beginning to work together. With short, fast intervals and hill runs (with limited rest between each) in our training schedule, working you aerobically and anaerobically, we continue down that path toward more economical, more forceful muscles.

This same schedule of runs hits a different kind of strength as well, one you may not have even thought of before: neuromuscular strength. Here we are not talking about the quality or the size of our muscles, but rather how well they're controlled. Specifically, you're training your nervous system to do a better job of recruiting and stimulating muscle fibers. The more signals you can send from your brain to your muscles, the more efficient they'll become. To put it another way, your nerves learn to activate your leg muscles more quickly and invite more muscle fibers to do so. Through this, you will have improved strength to scale the various climbs on a race course, as well as the power to climb those hills and mountains much quicker, with less fatigue.

Raw Speed

First let me tell you what I consider raw speed: the amount of distance you can cover running for one minute. A short, fast effort.

At first blush, you might think, raw speed . . . that is not a concern of a distance runner. For the recreational runner, particularly a beginning one, speed rarely fits into their calculations. They simply want to finish that 10K, half, or marathon, without collapsing into a pool of sweat and pain. I get it.

Then there are many others who think raw speed is really an innate talent. They're as fast as they're going to be. Yes and no. Yes, given perfect form, conditioning, you definitely have a physical limit to how fast you can run two hundred meters. No, you are probably not at that physical limit at this moment. In other words, there's room for improvement.

Raw speed dictates your ability and potential performance. The faster your raw speed, the faster you'll be across the board in race distances. Because they're cumulative, small improvements in raw speed are huge. In your upcoming training, you will do lots of short, fast interval runs on flat ground, which stress your anaerobic abilities. After a while, let's say you improve your two-hundred-meter time by three seconds. That translates to roughly twenty-four seconds off your minute-per-mile pace—a big improvement on your ability and potential.

Finally, short, fast efforts simply feel good to do. They improve your range of motion. They produce chemicals in the body that act like lubrication. In other words, fast, fun speed runs make your body feel good and healthy.

The Mix

In some stages of building your foundation, we will focus on primarily training one of the three key ingredients in your mix: endurance, strength, or speed. Yet at other stages, we will concentrate on endurance and its different forms—looking to train in strength endurance (how long you can maintain the force on your muscles) and speed endurance (how long you can maintain a certain speed). I hope you have the basic idea. Your body is a beautifully complicated beast; we're trying to work every bit of it to run well long.

The Game of Running—Tarahumara Indians

We've already talked a lot about how the Tarahumara lifestyle helps them to be the natural-born ultramarathon runners they are. What is a mystery to many—how to train to maximize our running ability and performance—the Tarahumara do as part of their daily life. Yes, they have great strength and form, but they also have a lifestyle from childhood forward that gives them a natural base of speed, strength, and endurance.

From the time Tarahumara children take their first steps, they're walking a lot, all the time, up and down hills. No horses, no cars, no buses, no bikes. If they want to get somewhere, they hoof it. And they love running!

But if you had to call one thing they do the "secret weapon" of their culture, it would have to be the game rarajípari. Children play as soon as they can (though at shorter distances than the adults). Here's the game: Take eight to ten players per team and an agreed-upon distance for the race, usually 5 to 10K for their kids on an out-and-back course (so the village can watch). The objective is to be the first team to kick a baseball-size wooden ball over the race distance. Some players carry a short stick to roll the ball on top of their foot to flick it really high, but otherwise it's a ball and some very fast feet moving all the time over hilly, uneven terrain. With short, fast runs up and down the canyons, chasing after a ball, Tarahumara children develop incredible speed and strength—and have fun doing it.

By adulthood, the Tarahumara easily transition to the longer fifty-to-a-hundred-mile version of the game. At this point, they need very little, if any, additional training to compete at the much advanced adult race distance and win ultramarathons.

THE FOUNDATION PROGRAM

Preparation Phase

Before even beginning this preparation phase, you will want to have finished the performance running transition, acclimating your body to the new demands of proper run form. Further, you've hopefully been working on your strength training.

Prior to launching into the heart of the foundation program, you also need to build up a base level of fitness. Now that your calves have stopped burning and your glutes are firing well, you'll want to work on building some consistency and endurance to prepare yourself for the demands of the foundation program. For those veteran runners who already feel they have a solid base, consider this preparation phase a time to continue your rejuvenation and focus on run form. (Resist the urge to do more; you'll be working plenty soon enough!)

Schedule

Continue with your strength training and do four thirty-minute easy runs per week for three to six weeks (or longer if you want) before starting the run foundation program. These runs should continue to be a low-intensity effort. Work on your forefoot strike and good form awareness. Proper run form is a lifelong pursuit—and if you want, feel free to continue working the run form drills during this preparation phase.

Here we are. Halfway around the lake. Follow me up on this boulder. Easy now as we get to the edge. It's a thirty-foot drop to the water. This is Jumping Rock, aptly named, since swimmers leap off it into the lake. Don't be fooled by the summer air, though. That water is freezing, even now, but what a great way to soak those sore calves.

The Jumping Rock is the perfect metaphor for where you are now. Time to leap into a new kind of running program, one designed specifically for you.

I know there are all kinds of training schedules out there. Do this many miles today, that many tomorrow, a total number this week; increase as you progress; then taper off a few weeks before race day. Some add interval runs and hill work. Some include cross-training. Many are quite useful in pursuing specific race distances, and you may want to follow them after you work this program.

But first things first. Work this five-month program. You'll build a strong, enduring base from which you can do any type of running you want.

After the preparation phase I outlined for you, you begin the foundation program by establishing your current level of fitness. To do that, we'll embark on two tests that measure where you are today in your ingredient mix. With these results, we can establish the training zones (based on heart rate and speed) you should be working at throughout different parts of the five-month program. On most runs, you'll be monitoring your heart rate or speed in order to maintain certain efforts specific to the purpose of that day.

The program is both customized and strategic. You begin from where you are in terms of strength, speed, and endurance. You're always training to your level of ability, and through monitoring each run, you're realizing the purpose of each workout, whether it's endurance, strength, speed, or a blend of two or all three. No undertraining, no overtraining. Maximum benefit for your effort.

Central to realizing this maximum benefit is the idea of thresholds. I believe that in every part of your mix—strength, endurance, speed, or combinations thereof—there is a certain level of sustained, steady effort (based on length of time and speed/intensity) that you are able to maintain without breaking down or realizing diminishing returns. By continuously working to these levels (through the training zones in your schedule), you get as much bang for your buck as possible. This works across the intensity spectrum, from thresholds of fat-burning runs to fast intervals to improve speed endurance.

There are two distinct phases in the five-month program. Cleverly, I'll call them phase one and phase two. You'll see them indicated in your schedule.

In phase one, we aim primarily to develop a solid base of your raw ingredients: aerobic endurance (cardiovascular, fat-burning efficiency), strength (musculoskeletal and neuromuscular), and raw speed. We progressively raise your volume of running in this phase. In phase two, we focus on higher-intensity workouts, really raising the bar on your anaerobic abilities in order to develop your speed endurance and strength endurance. The volume of running remains static, and in fact, we lower the time of your long runs. Over both phases of the program, we follow a stair-step schedule: three weeks of increasing effort, followed by one week of recovery.

Once you're finished with this program, once you have the foundation, you'll be a strong runner across the board. For the newbie, you can use this program to prepare for everything from a 5K to a half marathon. You'll be ready straightaway. You'll also likely do well in a marathon, but with a little more training, specifically some longer runs and marathon-pace runs, you're sure to cross that finish strong and fast.

For the veteran, take up this program after the season; use it to develop a new base on which to follow up with your own specific training/race goals. For the ultrarunner, follow this program to start your season and then do eight to ten weeks of longer, race-specific training runs leading into your race. See how much strength and speed improvement you find.

Equipment

First things first: You'll need to hit the stores to buy a GPS watch with a heart-rate monitor. If you don't have this already, it's a must. Consider me brand agnostic, but go for quality here. We want accuracy and reliability, so we know exactly how fast you're running in real time and what your heart rate is.

Test Phase

Once you've bought your equipment, we need to measure your current fitness with two distinct tests to identify your specific training zones. But some advice first: When you do these tests, don't absolutely kill yourself. This is not a competition. Do your best and understand that this is a benchmark test. As a coach, I'm looking to get a comment from an athlete after these tests something like, "I did well, but I think I can do better." That means you tried hard, but you weren't left sprawled on the track, cursing me.

When you do these tests, you'll want a flat, even surface. If there's a local high school or college track you can use, that would be perfect. If you can't get to a track, be sure to mark your course so you can replicate it for future tests.

Perform these two tests with two to three days of recovery between them. You can also run light and easy on the intervening days; just remember to be fresh for the tests. Also, before you do the test, be sure to do a practice run with your new watch so you know how to operate all the functions needed to record your data. It's never fun to repeat a test.

A. TEST ONE—ONE-MILE RUN

1. Warm-up: 20 minutes of easy running; increase to moderate pace for the last 5 minutes. Then do 4 short bursts of speed (or pickups) for roughly 30 seconds each (building your speed throughout their duration), with 1 minute of rest (either easy running or walking, whichever feels better for you) between each. After the final pickup, take a minute or so of rest before the test. Remember: You do not need to record any HR/speed information during the warm-up.
2. Test: A timed one-mile run, executed as fast and as steadily as you can. Remember to start your watch to

measure your HR and speed at the beginning of this test and to stop your watch at the end, so you capture only the test portion of your run.
3. Cooldown: 10 minutes of slow, easy running or walking.
4. Data: Record your average HR and max HR and total time for the test.

B. TEST TWO—20-MINUTE RUN

1. Warm-up: 15 minutes of easy running; increase to moderate pace for the last 5 minutes. Then do 4 short bursts of speed (or pickups) for roughly 30 seconds each (building your speed throughout their duration), with one minute of rest between each. After the final pickup, take a minute or so of rest before the test. Remember: You do not need to record any HR/speed information during the warm-up.
2. Test: A 20-minute run, executed as fast and as steadily as you can. Remember to start your watch to measure your HR and speed at the beginning of this test and stop your watch at the end, so you capture only the test portion of your run.
3. Cooldown: 10 minutes of slow, easy running or walking.
4. Data: Record your average HR and max HR, your average minute-per-mile speed, and the distance run during the test.

C. JUST-FOR-FUN TEST—ONE-MINUTE RUN

1. Warm-up: 20 minutes of easy running; increase to moderate pace for the last 5 minutes. Then do 4 short bursts of speed (or pickups) for roughly 30 seconds each (building your speed throughout their duration), with one minute of rest between each. After final pickup, take

a minute or so of rest before the test. Remember: You do not need to record any HR/speed information during the warm-up.

2. Test: A one-minute run, executed as fast as you can. Remember to start your watch to measure your speed and distance at the beginning of this test and stop your watch at the end, so you capture only the test portion of your run.
3. Cooldown: 10 minutes of slow, easy running or walking.
4. Data: Record your average speed and distance for this test.

Training Zones

Once you perform the tests, you'll have the data you need to establish your heart rate and speed zones. You will then use these zones in the training schedule to determine how fast or at what heart rate you will execute the daily workouts throughout the five-month program. Again, it's strategic because these workouts are based on your current fitness level, so that we are maximizing your gains in strength, speed, and endurance, while avoiding over- or undertraining. This is not a one-size-fits-all program. Quite the opposite.

Now to determine your speed zones (SP zones), take your one-mile test time and match it with the one closest to yours on the left-hand column of the SP zone chart below. If it's not exact, round to the closest time listed. Then run your finger straight to the right on the chart to see where your speed zone is on the list of 1 to 7. As an example, if your one-mile test time was 7:57, you would round down to the 7:55 time on the left-hand column of the chart. Then your SP zone 1 time range would be 11:12 to 10:41. This means that you should run workouts specified to be performed at the SP zone 1 level at a pace between 11:12 and 10:41 per mile. Your SP zone 5 range would be 8:34 to 8:18 per mile, and therefore you would run workouts specified in this zone at a minute-per-mile pace within that range. You will use all seven SP zones in your program.

ONE MILE TEST TIME	SP ZONE 1		SP ZONE 2		SP ZONE 3		SP ZONE 4		SP ZONE 5		SP ZONE 6		SP ZONE 7	
10:00	14:01	13:30	12:31	12:00	12:00	11:30	11:20	11:00	10:45	10:30	10:15	10:00	9:40	9:30
9:55	13:54	13:23	12:25	11:54	11:54	11:24	11:14	10:54	10:40	10:24	10:10	9:55	9:35	9:25
9:50	13:48	13:16	12:19	11:48	11:48	11:18	11:09	10:49	10:35	10:19	10:05	9:50	9:30	9:20
9:45	13:41	13:09	12:13	11:42	11:42	11:12	11:03	10:43	10:30	10:14	10:00	9:45	9:25	9:15
9:40	13:34	13:03	12:07	11:36	11:36	11:07	10:58	10:38	10:24	10:09	9:55	9:40	9:21	9:11
9:35	13:27	12:56	12:01	11:30	11:30	11:01	10:52	10:32	10:19	10:03	9:50	9:35	9:16	9:06
9:30	13:21	12:49	11:55	11:24	11:24	10:55	10:47	10:27	10:14	9:58	9:45	9:30	9:11	9:01
9:25	13:14	12:42	11:49	11:18	11:18	10:49	10:41	10:21	10:09	9:53	9:40	9:25	9:06	8:56
9:20	13:07	12:36	11:43	11:12	11:12	10:44	10:36	10:16	10:03	9:48	9:35	9:20	9:02	8:52
9:15	13:00	12:29	11:37	11:06	11:06	10:38	10:30	10:10	9:58	9:42	9:30	9:15	8:57	8:47
9:10	12:54	12:22	11:31	11:00	11:00	10:32	10:25	10:05	9:53	9:37	9:25	9:10	8:52	8:42
9:05	12:47	12:15	11:25	10:54	10:54	10:26	10:19	9:59	9:48	9:32	9:20	9:05	8:47	8:37
9:00	12:40	12:09	11:19	10:48	10:48	10:21	10:14	9:54	9:42	9:27	9:15	9:00	8:43	8:33
8:55	12:33	12:02	11:13	10:42	10:42	10:15	10:08	9:48	9:37	9:21	9:10	8:55	8:38	8:28
8:50	12:27	11:55	11:07	10:36	10:36	10:09	10:03	9:43	9:32	9:16	9:05	8:50	8:33	8:23
8:45	12:20	11:48	11:01	10:30	10:30	10:03	9:57	9:37	9:27	9:11	9:00	8:45	8:28	8:18
8:40	12:13	11:42	10:55	10:24	10:24	9:58	9:52	9:32	9:21	9:06	8:55	8:40	8:24	8:14
8:35	12:06	11:35	10:49	10:18	10:18	9:52	9:46	9:26	9:16	9:00	8:50	8:35	8:19	8:09

ONE MILE TEST TIME	SP ZONE 1		SP ZONE 2		SP ZONE 3		SP ZONE 4		SP ZONE 5		SP ZONE 6		SP ZONE 7	
8:30	12:00	11:28	10:43	10:12	10:12	9:46	9:41	9:21	9:11	8:55	8:45	8:30	8:14	8:04
8:25	11:53	11:21	10:37	10:06	10:06	9:40	9:35	9:15	9:06	8:50	8:40	8:25	8:09	7:59
8:20	11:46	11:15	10:31	10:00	10:00	9:35	9:30	9:10	9:00	8:45	8:35	8:20	8:05	7:55
8:15	11:39	11:08	10:25	9:54	9:54	9:29	9:24	9:04	8:55	8:39	8:30	8:15	8:00	7:50
8:10	11:33	11:01	10:19	9:48	9:48	9:23	9:19	8:59	8:50	8:34	8:25	8:10	7:55	7:45
8:05	11:26	10:54	10:13	9:42	9:42	9:17	9:13	8:53	8:45	8:29	8:20	8:05	7:50	7:40
8:00	11:19	10:48	10:07	9:36	9:36	9:12	9:08	8:48	8:39	8:24	8:15	8:00	7:46	7:36
7:55	11:12	10:41	10:01	9:30	9:30	9:06	9:02	8:42	8:34	8:18	8:10	7:55	7:41	7:31
7:50	11:06	10:34	9:55	9:24	9:24	9:00	8:57	8:37	8:29	8:13	8:05	7:50	7:36	7:26
7:45	10:59	10:27	9:49	9:18	9:18	8:54	8:51	8:31	8:24	8:08	8:00	7:45	7:31	7:21
7:40	10:52	10:21	9:43	9:12	9:12	8:49	8:46	8:26	8:18	8:03	7:55	7:40	7:27	7:17
7:35	10:45	10:14	9:37	9:06	9:06	8:43	8:40	8:20	8:13	7:57	7:50	7:35	7:22	7:12
7:30	10:39	10:07	9:31	9:00	9:00	8:37	8:35	8:15	8:08	7:52	7:45	7:30	7:17	7:07
7:25	10:32	10:00	9:25	8:54	8:54	8:31	8:29	8:09	8:03	7:47	7:40	7:25	7:12	7:02
7:20	10:25	9:54	9:19	8:48	8:48	8:26	8:24	8:04	7:57	7:42	7:35	7:20	7:08	6:58
7:15	10:18	9:47	9:13	8:42	8:42	8:20	8:18	7:58	7:52	7:36	7:30	7:15	7:03	6:53
7:10	10:12	9:40	9:07	8:36	8:36	8:14	8:13	7:53	7:47	7:31	7:25	7:10	6:58	6:48
7:05	10:05	9:33	9:01	8:30	8:30	8:08	8:07	7:47	7:42	7:26	7:20	7:05	6:53	6:43

ONE MILE TEST TIME	SP ZONE 1		SP ZONE 2		SP ZONE 3		SP ZONE 4		SP ZONE 5		SP ZONE 6		SP ZONE 7	
7:00	9:58	9:27	8:55	8:24	8:24	8:03	8:02	7:42	7:36	7:21	7:15	7:00	6:49	6:39
6:58	9:55	9:24	8:53	8:21	8:21	8:00	7:59	7:39	7:34	7:18	7:13	6:58	6:47	6:37
6:55	9:51	9:20	8:49	8:18	8:18	7:57	7:56	7:36	7:31	7:15	7:10	6:55	6:44	6:34
6:53	9:49	9:17	8:47	8:15	8:15	7:54	7:54	7:34	7:29	7:13	7:08	6:53	6:42	6:32
6:50	9:45	9:13	8:43	8:12	8:12	7:51	7:51	7:31	7:26	7:10	7:05	6:50	6:39	6:29
6:48	9:42	9:10	8:41	8:09	8:09	7:49	7:48	7:28	7:24	7:08	7:03	6:48	6:37	6:27
6:45	9:38	9:06	8:37	8:06	8:06	7:45	7:45	7:25	7:21	7:05	7:00	6:45	6:34	6:24
6:43	9:35	9:04	8:35	8:03	8:03	7:43	7:43	7:23	7:18	7:03	6:58	6:43	6:32	6:22
6:40	9:31	9:00	8:31	8:00	8:00	7:40	7:40	7:20	7:15	7:00	6:55	6:40	6:30	6:20
6:38	9:28	8:57	8:29	7:57	7:57	7:37	7:37	7:17	7:13	6:57	6:53	6:38	6:28	6:18
6:35	9:24	8:53	8:25	7:54	7:54	7:34	7:34	7:14	7:10	6:54	6:50	6:35	6:25	6:15
6:33	9:22	8:50	8:23	7:51	7:51	7:31	7:32	7:12	7:08	6:52	6:48	6:33	6:23	6:13
6:30	9:18	8:46	8:19	7:48	7:48	7:28	7:29	7:09	7:05	6:49	6:45	6:30	6:20	6:10
6:28	9:15	8:43	8:17	7:45	7:45	7:26	7:26	7:06	7:03	6:47	6:43	6:28	6:18	6:08
6:25	9:11	8:39	8:13	7:42	7:42	7:22	7:23	7:03	7:00	6:44	6:40	6:25	6:15	6:05
6:23	9:08	8:37	8:11	7:39	7:39	7:20	7:21	7:01	6:57	6:42	6:38	6:23	6:13	6:03
6:20	9:04	8:33	8:07	7:36	7:36	7:17	7:18	6:58	6:54	6:39	6:35	6:20	6:11	6:01
6:18	9:01	8:30	8:05	7:33	7:33	7:14	7:15	6:55	6:52	6:36	6:33	6:18	6:09	5:59

ONE MILE TEST TIME	SP ZONE 1		SP ZONE 2		SP ZONE 3		SP ZONE 4		SP ZONE 5		SP ZONE 6		SP ZONE 7	
6:15	8:57	8:26	8:01	7:30	7:30	7:11	7:12	6:52	6:49	6:33	6:30	6:15	6:06	5:56
6:13	8:55	8:23	7:59	7:27	7:27	7:08	7:10	6:50	6:47	6:31	6:28	6:13	6:04	5:54
6:10	8:51	8:19	7:55	7:24	7:24	7:05	7:07	6:47	6:44	6:28	6:25	6:10	6:01	5:51
6:08	8:48	8:16	7:53	7:21	7:21	7:03	7:04	6:44	6:42	6:26	6:23	6:08	5:59	5:49
6:05	8:44	8:12	7:49	7:18	7:18	6:59	7:01	6:41	6:39	6:23	6:20	6:05	5:56	5:46
6:03	8:41	8:10	7:47	7:15	7:15	6:57	6:59	6:39	6:36	6:21	6:18	6:03	5:54	5:44
6:00	8:37	8:06	7:43	7:12	7:12	6:54	6:56	6:36	6:33	6:18	6:15	6:00	5:52	5:42
5:58	8:34	8:03	7:41	7:09	7:09	6:51	6:53	6:33	6:31	6:15	6:13	5:58	5:50	5:40
5:55	8:30	7:59	7:37	7:06	7:06	6:48	6:50	6:30	6:28	6:12	6:10	5:55	5:47	5:37
5:53	8:28	7:56	7:35	7:03	7:03	6:45	6:48	6:28	6:26	6:10	6:08	5:53	5:45	5:35
5:50	8:24	7:52	7:31	7:00	7:00	6:42	6:45	6:25	6:23	6:07	6:05	5:50	5:42	5:32
5:48	8:21	7:49	7:29	6:57	6:57	6:40	6:42	6:22	6:21	6:05	6:03	5:48	5:40	5:30
5:45	8:17	7:45	7:25	6:54	6:54	6:36	6:39	6:19	6:18	6:02	6:00	5:45	5:37	5:27
5:43	8:14	7:43	7:23	6:51	6:51	6:34	6:37	6:17	6:15	6:00	5:58	5:43	5:35	5:25
5:40	8:10	7:39	7:19	6:48	6:48	6:31	6:34	6:14	6:12	5:57	5:55	5:40	5:33	5:23
5:38	8:07	7:36	7:17	6:45	6:45	6:28	6:31	6:11	6:10	5:54	5:53	5:38	5:31	5:21
5:35	8:03	7:32	7:13	6:42	6:42	6:25	6:28	6:08	6:07	5:51	5:50	5:35	5:28	5:18
5:33	8:01	7:29	7:11	6:39	6:39	6:22	6:26	6:06	6:05	5:49	5:48	5:33	5:26	5:16

ONE MILE TEST TIME	SP ZONE 1		SP ZONE 2		SP ZONE 3		SP ZONE 4		SP ZONE 5		SP ZONE 6		SP ZONE 7	
5:30	7:57	7:25	7:07	6:36	6:36	6:19	6:23	6:03	6:02	5:46	5:45	5:30	5:23	5:13
5:28	7:54	7:22	7:05	6:33	6:33	6:17	6:20	6:00	6:00	5:44	5:43	5:28	5:21	5:11
5:25	7:50	7:18	7:01	6:30	6:30	6:13	6:17	5:57	5:57	5:41	5:40	5:25	5:18	5:08
5:23	7:47	7:16	6:59	6:27	6:27	6:11	6:15	5:55	5:54	5:39	5:38	5:23	5:16	5:06
5:20	7:43	7:12	6:55	6:24	6:24	6:08	6:12	5:52	5:51	5:36	5:35	5:20	5:14	5:04
5:18	7:40	7:09	6:53	6:21	6:21	6:05	6:09	5:49	5:49	5:33	5:33	5:18	5:12	5:02
5:15	7:36	7:05	6:49	6:18	6:18	6:02	6:06	5:46	5:46	5:30	5:30	5:15	5:09	4:59
5:13	7:34	7:02	6:47	6:15	6:15	5:59	6:04	5:44	5:44	5:28	5:28	5:13	5:07	4:57
5:10	7:30	6:58	6:43	6:12	6:12	5:56	6:01	5:41	5:41	5:25	5:25	5:10	5:04	4:54
5:08	7:27	6:55	6:41	6:09	6:09	5:54	5:58	5:38	5:39	5:23	5:23	5:08	5:02	4:52
5:05	7:23	6:51	6:37	6:06	6:06	5:50	5:55	5:35	5:36	5:20	5:20	5:05	4:59	4:49
5:03	7:20	6:49	6:35	6:03	6:03	5:48	5:53	5:33	5:33	5:18	5:18	5:03	4:57	4:47
5:00	7:16	6:45	6:31	6:00	6:00	5:45	5:50	5:30	5:30	5:15	5:15	5:00	4:55	4:45
4:58	7:13	6:42	6:29	5:57	5:57	5:42	5:47	5:27	5:28	5:12	5:13	4:58	4:53	4:43
4:55	7:09	6:38	6:25	5:54	5:54	5:39	5:44	5:24	5:25	5:09	5:10	4:55	4:50	4:40
4:53	7:07	6:35	6:23	5:51	5:51	5:36	5:42	5:22	5:23	5:07	5:08	4:53	4:48	4:38
4:50	7:03	6:31	6:19	5:48	5:48	5:33	5:39	5:19	5:20	5:04	5:05	4:50	4:45	4:35
4:48	7:00	6:28	6:17	5:45	5:45	5:31	5:36	5:16	5:18	5:02	5:03	4:48	4:43	4:33

ONE MILE TEST TIME	SP ZONE 1		SP ZONE 2		SP ZONE 3		SP ZONE 4		SP ZONE 5		SP ZONE 6		SP ZONE 7	
4:45	6:56	6:24	6:13	5:42	5:42	5:27	5:33	5:13	5:15	4:59	5:00	4:45	4:40	4:30
4:43	6:53	6:22	6:11	5:39	5:39	5:25	5:31	5:11	5:12	4:57	4:58	4:43	4:38	4:28
4:40	6:49	6:18	6:07	5:36	5:36	5:22	5:28	5:08	5:09	4:54	4:55	4:40	4:36	4:26
4:38	6:46	6:15	6:05	5:33	5:33	5:19	5:25	5:05	5:07	4:51	4:53	4:38	4:34	4:24
4:35	6:42	6:11	6:01	5:30	5:30	5:16	5:22	5:02	5:04	4:48	4:50	4:35	4:31	4:21
4:33	6:40	6:08	5:59	5:27	5:27	5:13	5:20	5:00	5:02	4:46	4:48	4:33	4:29	4:19
4:30	6:36	6:04	5:55	5:24	5:24	5:10	5:17	4:57	4:59	4:43	4:45	4:30	4:26	4:16
4:28	6:33	6:01	5:53	5:21	5:21	5:08	5:14	4:54	4:57	4:41	4:43	4:28	4:24	4:14
4:25	6:29	5:57	5:49	5:18	5:18	5:04	5:11	4:51	4:54	4:38	4:40	4:25	4:21	4:11
4:23	6:26	5:55	5:47	5:15	5:15	5:02	5:09	4:49	4:51	4:36	4:38	4:23	4:19	4:09
4:20	6:22	5:51	5:43	5:12	5:12	4:59	5:06	4:46	4:48	4:33	4:35	4:20	4:17	4:07
4:18	6:19	5:48	5:41	5:09	5:09	4:56	5:03	4:43	4:46	4:30	4:33	4:18	4:15	4:05
4:15	6:15	5:44	5:37	5:06	5:06	4:53	5:00	4:40	4:43	4:27	4:30	4:15	4:12	4:02
4:13	6:13	5:41	5:35	5:03	5:03	4:50	4:58	4:38	4:41	4:25	4:28	4:13	4:10	4:00
4:10	6:09	5:37	5:31	5:00	5:00	4:47	4:55	4:35	4:38	4:22	4:25	4:10	4:07	3:57
4:08	6:06	5:34	5:29	4:57	4:57	4:45	4:52	4:32	4:36	4:20	4:23	4:08	4:05	3:55
4:05	6:02	5:30	5:25	4:54	4:54	4:41	4:49	4:29	4:33	4:17	4:20	4:05	4:02	3:52
4:03	5:59	5:28	5:23	4:51	4:51	4:39	4:47	4:27	4:30	4:15	4:18	4:03	4:00	3:50

ONE MILE TEST TIME	SP ZONE 1		SP ZONE 2		SP ZONE 3		SP ZONE 4		SP ZONE 5		SP ZONE 6		SP ZONE 7	
4:00	5:55	5:24	5:19	4:48	4:48	4:36	4:44	4:24	4:27	4:12	4:15	4:00	3:58	3:48
3:58	5:52	5:21	5:17	4:45	4:45	4:33	4:41	4:21	4:25	4:09	4:13	3:58	3:56	3:46
3:55	5:48	5:17	5:13	4:42	4:42	4:30	4:38	4:18	4:22	4:06	4:10	3:55	3:53	3:43
3:50	5:42	5:10	5:07	4:36	4:36	4:24	4:33	4:13	4:17	4:01	4:05	3:50	3:48	3:38
3:48	5:39	5:07	5:05	4:33	4:33	4:22	4:30	4:10	4:15	3:59	4:03	3:48	3:46	3:36
3:45	5:35	5:03	5:01	4:30	4:30	4:18	4:27	4:07	4:12	3:56	4:00	3:45	3:43	3:33

* Speed Zones are in minute-per-mile pace

To determine your heart rate zones (HR zones), take your average heart rate (avg. HR) during the 20-minute test run and match it with the avg. HR number in the left-hand column of the HR zone chart on the next page. Then run your finger straight to the right on the chart to see your HR zones, 1 to 7. As an example, if your 20-minute test run avg. HR was 165, then your HR zone 2 range would be 133 to 142. This means that you should run workouts specified to be performed at HR zone 2 level with an effort that brings your monitored heart rate to between 133 and 142 beats per minute. Your HR zone 7 level, your most intense HR zone workout, would then require you to bring your average heart rate to between 161 and 165 beats per minute. You will use all seven HR zones in your program.

TEST AVG HEART RATE	HR ZONE 1		HR ZONE 2		HR ZONE 3		HR ZONE 4		HR ZONE 5		HR ZONE 6		HR ZONE 7	
150	108	117	118	127	128	132	133	136	137	141	142	145	146	150
151	109	118	119	128	129	133	134	137	138	142	143	146	147	151
152	110	119	120	129	130	134	135	138	139	143	144	147	148	152
153	111	120	121	130	131	135	136	139	140	144	145	148	149	153
154	112	121	122	131	132	136	137	140	141	145	146	149	150	154
155	113	122	123	132	133	137	138	141	142	146	147	150	151	155
156	114	123	124	133	134	138	139	142	143	147	148	151	152	156
157	115	124	125	134	135	139	140	143	144	148	149	152	153	157
158	116	125	126	135	136	140	141	144	145	149	150	153	154	158
159	117	126	127	136	137	141	142	145	146	150	151	154	155	159
160	118	127	128	137	138	142	143	146	147	151	152	155	156	160
161	119	128	129	138	139	143	144	147	148	152	153	156	157	161
162	120	129	130	139	140	144	145	148	149	153	154	157	158	162
163	121	130	131	140	141	145	146	149	150	154	155	158	159	163
164	122	131	132	141	142	146	147	150	151	155	156	159	160	164
165	123	132	133	142	143	147	148	151	152	156	157	160	161	165
166	124	133	134	143	144	148	149	152	153	157	158	161	162	166
167	125	134	135	144	145	149	150	153	154	158	159	162	163	167

TEST AVG HEART RATE	HR ZONE 1		HR ZONE 2		HR ZONE 3		HR ZONE 4		HR ZONE 5		HR ZONE 6		HR ZONE 7	
168	126	135	136	145	146	150	151	154	155	159	160	163	164	168
169	127	136	137	146	147	151	152	155	156	160	161	164	165	169
170	128	137	138	147	148	152	153	156	157	161	162	165	166	170
171	129	138	139	148	149	153	154	157	158	162	163	166	167	171
172	130	139	140	149	150	154	155	158	159	163	164	167	168	172
173	131	140	141	150	151	155	156	159	160	164	165	168	169	173
174	132	141	142	151	152	156	157	160	161	165	166	169	170	174
175	133	142	143	152	153	157	158	161	162	166	167	170	171	175
176	134	143	144	153	154	158	159	162	163	167	168	171	172	176
177	135	144	145	154	155	159	160	163	164	168	169	172	173	177
178	136	145	146	155	156	160	161	164	165	169	170	173	174	178
179	137	146	147	156	157	161	162	165	166	170	171	174	175	179
180	138	147	148	157	158	162	163	166	167	171	172	175	176	180
181	139	148	149	158	159	163	164	167	168	172	173	176	177	181
182	140	149	150	159	160	164	165	168	169	173	174	177	178	182
183	141	150	151	160	161	165	166	169	170	174	175	178	179	183
184	142	151	152	161	162	166	167	170	171	175	176	179	180	184
185	143	152	153	162	163	167	168	171	172	176	177	180	181	185

TEST AVG HEART RATE	HR ZONE 1		HR ZONE 2		HR ZONE 3		HR ZONE 4		HR ZONE 5		HR ZONE 6		HR ZONE 7	
186	144	153	154	163	164	168	169	172	173	177	178	181	182	186
187	145	154	155	164	165	169	170	173	174	178	179	182	183	187
188	146	155	156	165	166	170	171	174	175	179	180	183	184	188
189	147	156	157	166	167	171	172	175	176	180	181	184	185	189
190	148	157	158	167	168	172	173	176	177	181	182	185	186	190
191	149	158	159	168	169	173	174	177	178	182	183	186	187	191
192	150	159	160	169	170	174	175	178	179	183	184	187	188	192
193	151	160	161	170	171	175	176	179	180	184	185	188	189	193
194	152	161	162	171	172	176	177	180	181	185	186	189	190	194
195	153	162	163	172	173	177	178	181	182	186	187	190	191	195
196	154	163	164	173	174	178	179	182	183	187	188	191	192	196
197	155	164	165	174	175	179	180	183	184	188	189	192	193	197
198	156	165	166	175	176	180	181	184	185	189	190	193	194	198
199	157	166	167	176	177	181	182	185	186	190	191	194	195	199
200	158	167	168	177	178	182	183	186	187	191	192	195	196	200

* Heart Rate zones are measured in beats per minute

Now, how do I calculate these zones? The specific calculations weave in a whole bunch of physiological science, not to mention knowledge I've won in seeing how far and how fast to push athletes. It's likely I could write a whole book on these zones, but the truth is that you don't need the science behind the zones for the program to benefit you. Simply put: The zones help accomplish the overall outcome and purpose of the program.

Still, it's nice to know what you'll be getting from each zone in terms of effort and benefit. I've given you the broad strokes, plus some helpful tips for each below. As part of this, I throw out some terms that need some brief explanation so you're clear on what I mean.

- *Aerobic effort*—This refers to an easy to moderately paced run. Your energy is produced with the use of oxygen.
- *Anaerobic effort*—Typically, short, fast, and intense runs, like sprints. You're working really hard in this kind of exercise, and your energy is being produced without oxygen.
- *VO2max*—The maximum rate at which oxygen is consumed in your body. This is basically a measure of your aerobic capacity, or, as I like to put it, it's a measure of how big and efficient your engine is.
- *Threshold*—You may have heard of a lactate threshold, which is a measure of how fast you can go while still using oxygen to create fuel. You go over it, you feel that burn (lactic acid) in your muscles, your breathing becomes noticeably labored, and you fatigue quickly.
- *Race-pace training*—In the zones, you will see me refer to "marathon training heart rate effort" or "10K training speed pace." This is often the nomenclature you'll see used in other running schedules. I use it here to give you reference—and also if you want to use these training zones for specific race schedules after building your strategic foundation. Please note these pace efforts are to be used in training, not specifically in setting a race-pace expectation.

Okay, onward. Let me take a moment to explain what the different zones are for in the charts.

HEART RATE ZONES

HR Zone 1

Runs in this zone are for recovery from harder, longer workouts. Recovery is a vital part of training, and when your body rebuilds, you get stronger and faster. Runners often fail to understand the importance of these runs and often do them too hard. This zone is also used in warm-ups, cooldowns, and rest intervals.

Run this zone alone, so you are not tempted to pace too fast with friends. It should be run on flat terrain to keep your heart rate in the zone.

HR Zone 2

Many of your weekly miles will be performed in this zone. They will build the aerobic engine and provide the long-term foundation of economy and endurance for future faster running. This zone especially develops greater fat-burning efficiency. Now, remember: This is a slow run with a lot of purpose, even though it may be hard at first to maintain a pace that is under what you may be used to in your former training. We're multiplying those beautiful mitochondria, and you will get faster at this lower effort.

With the slow pace, the recovery time for these runs is limited, an added advantage. That means we can run more of them, more frequently. Finally, this zone allows us to focus on form and cadence.

Run this on flat to slightly rolling terrain, so you are able to manage effort and heart rate. Adjust duration to meet your ability and available training time that day.

HR Zone 3

A step up from zone 2, here you are beginning to develop some strength/muscle endurance, while continuing to build your aerobic engine and fat-burning abilities. Economy over long periods of time—that's where you're going.

Try to keep the terrain flat or rolling to maintain effort and heart rate, but this zone allows for more flexibility in pace to accompany friends or to hit a few low hills. Adjust duration to meet your ability and available training time.

HR Zone 4

Runs in this zone train for strength endurance, pushing you onto the edge of long, sustained, moderate aerobic efforts. They also prepare the body for even higher-intensity efforts.

Perform these runs on flat surfaces/low hills combined with occasional hilly trail runs. For reference to other training regimens (and those not using speed as the measure), this is a marathon training heart rate effort.

HR Zone 5

Now you are into the top end of your aerobic abilities, right under your lactate threshold. You are really developing strength endurance.

Keep good awareness and focus to stay within the small heart rate range of this zone. Be steady as you can throughout this run. Level terrain or long, steady hill climbs are the best. This is a half-marathon-training heart rate effort.

HR Zone 6

Runs in this zone are at your approximate aerobic threshold. You'll likely experience a change in breathing. There are potent benefits to training at this threshold: You're building muscle and speed endurance and increasing your ability to sustain faster, steadier efforts while remaining aerobic.

This is a 10K-training heart-rate effort.

HR Zone 7

In this zone, you are at your VO2max level, working your muscles to utilize a higher percentage of oxygen in your blood (improving efficiency) and bridging the gap between their aerobic/anaerobic capabilities (improving speed endurance).

This is a 5K-training heart rate effort.

SPEED ZONES

SP Zone 1

This is your endurance speed in minutes-per-mile pace, and runs in this zone help you sustain a consistent pace to build economy and efficiency.

SP Zone 2

Runs in this zone offer the same benefits as HR zone 4. This is your marathon-training pace in minutes per mile.

SP Zone 3

Runs in this zone offer the same benefits as HR zone 5. This is your half-marathon-training pace in minutes per mile.

SP Zone 4

Runs in this zone offer the same benefits as HR zone 6. This is your 10K-training pace in minutes per mile.

SP Zone 5

Runs in this zone offer the same benefits as HR zone 7. This is your 5K-training pace in minutes per mile.

SP Zone 6

Runs in this zone continue to push your aerobic capacity/VO2max in minutes-per-mile pace, again offering the same benefits as HR zone 7, but at shorter-duration intervals. For accurate exertion gauging, this speed zone is preferred over HR zone 7.

SP Zone 7

Used for speed intervals, runs in this zone train economy and focus on your anaerobic capabilities in minutes-per-mile pace. Your efforts here will help your neuromuscular development.

Execution Phase

Now that you know your heart rate and speed zones and have an understanding of their purpose, we can move on to the five-month training program. It requires discipline and awareness to execute, but if you follow through, you'll be amazed at your improved ability to run well, long, fast, and strong.

Here are some key glossary terms and examples of some of the shorthand terminology you'll need to know to follow the program.

- WU = warm-up
- MS = main set, core of the workout
- CD = cooldown
- RI = rest interval
- 10' = ten minutes

- 10" = ten seconds
- 15' in HRZ 2 = fifteen minutes of running in heart rate zone 2
- 4–6 X 2' at SPZ 4 w/2' RI = four to six interval runs for two minutes each in speed zone 4 range with a two-minute rest interval between each
- Asterisks are suggested optional days.

PHASE 1 — WEEK 1

Day 1

WU: 10' in HRZ 1–2.

MS: 20–45' steady running in HRZ 2 working on cadence. During this run perform a 10–20" moderately fast sprint every 5' throughout the run. Run by what feels moderately fast to you and then settle back into HRZ 2.

CD: 5' in HRZ 1.

***Day 2**

WU: 5–10' building to HRZ 2.

MS: 20–45' steady running in HRZ 2. Count your cadence every 5'. Count how many times your right foot strikes the ground in 15". Through time, aim for 22–23 per 15".

CD: 5' in HRZ 1.

DAY 3

WU: 15' in HRZ 1–3 + 4 × 30" building your speed to moderate fast by the end of each w/1' RI.

MS: 4–6 × 2' at SPZ 4 w/2' RI.

CD: 5' in HRZ 1.

***Day 4**

WU: 5–10' building to HRZ 2.

MS: 20–45' steady running in HRZ 2. Count your cadence every 5'. Count how many times your right foot strikes the ground in 15". Through time, aim for 22–23 per 15".

CD: 5' in HRZ 1.

Day 5

WU: 5' building to HRZ 2.

MS: 10–40' steady running in HRZ 2 and then finish run with 10' steady in SPZ 1.

CD: 5–10' in HRZ 1–2.

Day 6

WU: 5' building to HRZ 2.

MS: 30–65' steady in HRZ 2. Count your cadence every 5'. Today's run time should be 10–15' longer than your longest run in the last 2–3 weeks.

CD: 5' in HRZ 1.

Day 7: Day OFF

WU:

MS:

CD:

PHASE 1 - WEEK 2

Day 1

WU: 5–10' building to HRZ 2.

MS: 10–35' steady running in HRZ 2. Finishing run with 6 × 10" sprints w/1–2' walk RI. Look to build these sprints to faster than SPZ 7 pace.

CD: 5' in HRZ 1.

***Day 2**

WU: 5–10' building to HRZ 2.

MS: 20–45' steady running in HRZ 2. Count your cadence every 5'. Count how many times your right foot strikes the ground in 15". Through time, aim for 22–23 per 15".

CD: 5' in HRZ 1.

Day 3

WU: 15' in HRZ 1–2 + 4 × 30" building your speed to moderate fast by the end of each w/1' RI.

MS: 3–4 × 2' hill repeats at a strong and steady effort, but not max effort. Run by what feels moderately fast to you w/ 2–3' RI. Finish with 3–4 × 2' in SPZ 4 on flat terrain w/2' RI.

CD: 5' in HRZ 1.

***Day 4**

WU: 5' building to HRZ 2.

MS: 10–30' steady running in HRZ 2. Count your cadence every 5'.

CD: 5' in HRZ 1.

Day 5

WU: 15' slowly building HR to HRZ 3 by the end.

MS: 2–3 × 5' in HRZ 3 w/2' RI. Finish run with 5 × 20" moderately fast sprints w/1' RI.

CD: 5–10' in HRZ 1–2.

Day 6

WU: 5–10' building to HRZ 2.

MS: Long run steady in HRZ 2. Count your cadence every 5'. 10–15' longer than last week's long run.

CD: 5' in HRZ 1.

Day 7 Day OFF

WU:

MS:

CD:

PHASE 1 - WEEK 3

Day 1

WU: 10' in HRZ 1–2.

MS: 20–45' HRZ 2 running. During this run perform a 10–20" moderately fast sprint every 5' throughtout the run. Run by what feels moderately fast to you and then settle back into HRZ 2.

CD: 5' in HRZ 1.

***Day 2**

WU: 5–10' building to HRZ 2.

MS: 20–45' steady running in HRZ 2. Count your cadence every 5'. Count how many times your right foot strikes the ground in 15". Through time, aim for 22–23 per 15".

CD: 5' in HRZ 1.

Day 3

WU: 15' in HRZ 1–2 + 4 × 30" building your speed to moderate fast by the end of each w/1' RI.

MS: 6–8 × 2' at SPZ 4 w/2' RI.

CD: 5' in HRZ 1.

***Day 4**

WU: 5' in HRZ 1.

MS: Short recovery run in HRZ 1–2.

CD: 5' in HRZ 1.

Day 5

WU: 15' in HRZ 1–2 + 4 × 30" building your speed to moderate fast by the end of each w/1' RI.

MS: 3–5 × 1' at SPZ 6–7 w/1–2' RI. 3–5 × 30" sprints building your speed to faster than SPZ 7 by the end of each w/2' RI.

CD: 5' in HRZ 1.

Day 6

WU: 5–10' building to HRZ 2.

MS: Long run steady in HRZ 2. Be patient and resist the urge to go faster. 10–15' longer than last week's long run.

CD: 5' in HRZ 1.

Day 7 Day OFF

WU:

MS:

CD:

PHASE 1 - WEEK 4

Day 1

WU: 10' in HRZ 1–2.

MS: 15–30" steady running in HRZ 2. Count your cadence every 5'. Count how many times your right foot strikes the ground in 15". Through time, aim for 22–23 per 15".

CD: 5' in HRZ 1.

***Day 2**

WU: 5' in HRZ 1.

MS: Short recovery run in HRZ 1–2. This should be an OFF day if legs are tired, listen to your body.

CD: 5' in HRZ 1.

Day 3

WU: 15' in HRZ 1–2 + 4 × 30" building your speed to moderate fast by the end of each w/1' RI.

MS: 15–30' steady in SPZ 1.

CD: 5' in HRZ 1.

Day 4 Day OFF

WU:

MS:

CD:

Day 5

WU: 10' in HRZ 1–2.

MS: 15–30' steady HRZ 2 running working on cadence and form.

CD: 5' in HRZ 1.

Day 6

WU: 5–10' building to HRZ 2.

MS: Long run steady in HRZ 2. Do not increase your run time today. Keep it the same as your week 2 long run.

CD: 5' in HRZ 1.

Day 7 Day OFF

WU:

MS:

CD:

PHASE 1 - WEEK 5

Day 1

WU: 15' in HRZ 1–3 + 4 × 30" building your speed to moderate fast by the end of each w/1' RI.

MS: 3 × 5' in HRZ 5 w/2' RI.

CD: 5' in HRZ 1.

Day 2

WU: 15' in HRZ 1–3 + 4 × 30" building your speed to moderate fast by the end of each w/1' RI.

MS: 5–8 × 10" fast sprints w/1–2' RI. Run by what feels fast to you. Make it fun speed. If you dread these, they are too fast.

CD: 5' in HRZ 1.

***Day 3**

WU: 5–10' building to HRZ 2.

MS: 15–40' steady running in HRZ 2. Count your cadence every 5'.

CD: 5' in HRZ 1.

Day 4

WU: 15' in HRZ 1–2 + 4 × 30" building your speed to moderate fast by the end of each w/1' RI.

MS: 5–8 × 60–90" hill repeats at a strong and steady effort, but not max effort. Run by what feels moderately fast to you w/ 2–3' RI.

CD: 5' in HRZ 1.

***Day 5**

WU: 5–10' building to HRZ 2.

MS: 10–20' steady in HRZ 3.

CD: 5' in HRZ 1.

Day 6

WU: 5–10' building to HRZ 2.

MS: Long run steady HRZ 2 running working on cadence. Make this run 15' longer than week 3 long run.

CD: 5' in HRZ 1.

Day 7 Day OFF

WU:

MS:

CD:

PHASE 1 - WEEK 6

Day 1

WU: 5–10' building to HRZ 2.

MS: 20–45' steady running in HRZ 2. Count your cadence every 5'. Count how many times your right foot strikes the ground in 15". Through time, aim for 22–23 per 15".

CD: 5' in HRZ 1.

Day 2

WU: 15' in HRZ 1–3 + 4 × 30" building your speed to moderate fast by the end of each w/1' RI.

MS: 4 × 5' in HRZ 5 w/2' RI.

CD: 5' in HRZ 1.

***Day 3**

WU: 5' in HRZ 1.

MS: Short recovery run in HRZ 1–2. This should be an OFF day if legs are tired; listen to your body.

CD: 5' in HRZ 1.

Day 4

WU: 15' in HRZ 1–3 + 4 × 30" building your speed to moderate fast by the end of each w/1' RI.

MS: 4–5 × 10" fast sprints w/1–2' RI. Run by what feels fast to you. 4–6 × 1' at SPZ 7 w/2' RI.

CD: 5' in HRZ 1.

***Day 5**

WU: 5–10' building to HRZ 2.

MS: 10–30' steady running in HRZ 2. Count your cadence every 5'.

CD: 5' in HRZ 1.

Day 6

WU: 5–10' building to HRZ 2.

MS: Long run steady HRZ 2 with the last 15–30' in HRZ 3. Make this run 15' longer than week 5 long run.

CD: 5' in HRZ 1.

Day 7 Day OFF

WU:

MS:

CD:

PHASE 1 - WEEK 7

***Day 1**

WU: 5–10' building to HRZ 2.

MS: 20–45' steady running in HRZ 2. Count your cadence every 5'. Count how many times your right foot strikes the ground in 15". Through time, aim for 22–23 per 15".

CD: 5' in HRZ 1.

Day 2

WU: 10' in HRZ 1–2.

MS: 20–45' steady HRZ 2 running working on cadence. During this run perform a 10–20" moderately fast sprint every 5' throughtout the run. Run by what feels moderately fast to you and then settle back into HRZ 2.

CD: 5' in HRZ 1.

Day 3

WU: 15' in HRZ 1–3 + 4 × 30" building your speed to moderate fast by the end of each w/1' RI.

MS: 4–6 × 3' at SPZ 4 w/2' RI.

CD: 5' in HRZ 1.

***Day 4**

WU: 5–10' building to HRZ 2.

MS: 15–40' steady in HRZ 2. Count your cadence every 5'.

CD: 5' in HRZ 1.

Day 5

WU: 15' in HRZ 1–2 + 4 × 30" building your speed to moderate fast by the end of each w/1' RI.

MS: 6–10 × 60–90" hill repeats at a strong and steady effort, but not max effort. Run by what feels moderately fast to you w/ 2–3' RI.

CD: 5' in HRZ 1.

Day 6

WU: 5–10' building to HRZ 2.

MS: Long run in HRZ 2–3. Fluctuate effort as you feel. Make this run 15' longer than week 6 or no longer than 3 hours.

CD: 5' in HRZ 1.

Day 7 Day OFF

WU:

MS:

CD:

PHASE 1 - WEEK 8

***Day 1**

WU: 5–10' building to HRZ 2.

MS: 15–30' steady in HRZ 2. Count your cadence every 5'.

CD: 5' in HRZ 1.

Day 2 Day OFF

WU:

MS:

CD:

Day 3

WU: 5–10' building to HRZ 2.

MS: 20–45' in HRZ 2–3 as you feel.

CD: 5' in HRZ 1.

Day 4

WU: 5–10' building to HRZ 2.

MS: 20–40' at SPZ 1.

CD: 5' in HRZ 1.

Day 5 Day OFF

WU:

MS:

CD:

Day 6

WU: 5–10' building to HRZ 2.

MS: Long run steady in HRZ 2. Do not increase your run time today. Keep it the same as week 5 long run.

CD: 5' in HRZ 1.

Day 7 Day OFF

WU:

MS:

CD:

PHASE 1 - WEEK 9

Day 1

WU: 15' in HRZ 1–3 + 4 × 30" building your speed to moderate fast by the end of each w/1' RI.

MS: 3–4 × 8' steady in HRZ 5 w/3' RI.

CD: 5' in HRZ 1.

***Day 2**

WU: 5–10' building to HRZ 2.

MS: 15–40' steady in HRZ 2.

CD: 5' in HRZ 1.

Day 3

WU: 5–10' building to HRZ 2.

MS: HRZ 2–3. Finish with 5–6 × 10" sprints on flat or hills (mix it up) w/1' RI.

CD: 5' in HRZ 1.

Day 4

WU: 15' in HRZ 1–3 + 4 × 30" building your speed to moderate fast by the end of each w/1' RI.

MS: 4–6 × 4' in SPZ 4 w/3' RI.

CD: 5' in HRZ 1.

***Day 5**

WU: 5–10' building to HRZ 2.

MS: HRZ 1–2 recovery or day OFF.

CD: 5' in HRZ 1.

Day 6

WU: 5–10' building to HRZ 2.

MS: Long run in HRZ 2–3. Make this run 10–15' longer than week 7 or no longer than 3 hours.

CD: 5' in HRZ 1.

Day 7 Day OFF

WU:

MS:

CD:

PHASE 1 - WEEK 10

Day 1

WU: 5–10' building to HRZ 2.

MS: 15–40' in HRZ 2–3.

CD: 5' in HRZ 1.

Day 2

WU: 15' in HRZ 1–3 + 4 × 30" building your speed to moderate fast by the end of each w/1' RI.

MS: 4 × 5' in HRZ 5–6 w/3' RI.

CD: 5' in HRZ 1.

***Day 3**

WU: 5–10' building to HRZ 2.

MS: 15–40' steady in HRZ 2.

CD: 5' in HRZ 1.

Day 4

WU: 15' in HRZ 1–2 + 4 × 30" building your speed to moderate fast by the end of each w/1' RI.

MS: 4–5 × 2' hill repeats at a strong and steady effort. Run by feel, not HR, and use the downhill as an easy RI. 3–5 × 1' at SPZ 6–7 w/1–2' RI.

CD: 5' in HRZ 1.

***Day 5**

WU: 5–10' building to HRZ 2.

MS: Short recovery run in HRZ 1–2 or day OFF.

CD: 5' in HRZ 1.

Day 6

WU: 5–10' building to HRZ 2.

MS: Long run in HRZ 2–3 with the last 10–20' HRZ 4–5. Make this run the same length as week 9.

CD: 5' in HRZ 1.

Day 7 Day OFF

WU:

MS:

CD:

PHASE 1 - WEEK 11

Day 1

WU: 5–10' building to HRZ 2.

MS: 15–40' steady in HRZ 2.

CD: 5' in HRZ 1.

***Day 2**

WU: 5–10' building to HRZ 2.

MS: 15–40' steady in HRZ 2.

CD: 5' in HRZ 1.

Day 3

WU: 15' in HRZ 1–2 + 4 × 30" building your speed to moderate fast by the end of each w/1' RI.

MS: 4–6 × 4' in SPZ 4 w/3' RI.

CD: 5' in HRZ 1.

***Day 4**

WU: 5–10' building to HRZ 2.

MS: Short recovery run in HRZ 1–2 or day OFF.

CD: 5' in HRZ 1.

Day 5

WU: 15–30' in HRZ 1–3 + 4 × 30" building your speed to moderate fast by the end of each w/1' RI.

MS: 6–8 × 15–20" fast sprints w/2' RI.

CD: 5' in HRZ 1.

Day 6

WU: 5–10' building to HRZ 2.

MS: Long run in HRZ 2–3 with a 10" moderately fast pickup every 8–10' throughout the run. Make this run 15' longer than week 9 or no longer than 3 hours.

CD: 5' in HRZ 1.

Day 7 Day OFF

WU:

MS:

CD:

PHASE 1 - WEEK 12

Day 1 Day OFF

WU:

MS:

CD:

Day 2

WU: 20–25' in HRZ 1–3 + 4 × 30" building your speed to moderate fast by the end of each w/1' RI.

TEST: At the track, perform the same one-mile test that you did at the start of the program. Make adjustments to training zones before starting Phase 2.

CD: 5' in HRZ 1.

***Day 3**

WU: 5–10' building to HRZ 2.

MS: Short recovery run in HRZ 1–2 or day OFF.

CD: 5' in HRZ 1.

***Day 4**

WU: 5–10' building to HRZ 2.

MS: 15–30' steady in HRZ 2.

CD: 5' in HRZ 1.

Day 5

WU: 15' in HRZ 1–3 + 4 × 30" building your speed to moderate fast by the end of each w/1' RI.

TEST: At the track, perform the 20-minute test and make training zone adjustments before starting Phase 2.

CD: 5' in HRZ 1.

Day 6

WU: 5–10' building to HRZ 2.

MS: HRZ 2–3 as you feel. Make this run 50–60 percent shorter than your longest run in Phase 1.

CD: 5' in HRZ 1.

Day 7 Day OFF

WU:

MS:

CD:

PHASE 2 - WEEK 1

***Day 1**

WU: 10' in HRZ 1–2.

MS: 20–45' steady running in HRZ 2.

CD: 5' in HRZ 1.

Day 2

WU: 15' in HRZ 1–3 + 4 × 30" building your speed to moderate fast by the end of each w/1' RI.

MS: 3–5 × 3' at SPZ 6 w/3' RI.

CD: 5' in HRZ 1.

***Day 3**

WU: 5' in HRZ 1.

MS: Short recovery run in HRZ 1–2. Or Day OFF.

CD: 5' in HRZ 1.

Day 4

WU: 10' in HRZ 1–2.

MS: 15–40' steady running in HRZ 2. Finish with 5–8 × 10" sprints w/1' RI.

CD: 5' in HRZ 1.

Day 5

WU: 15' in HRZ 1–3 + 4 × 30" building your speed to moderate fast by the end of each w/1' RI.

MS: 20–30' in HRZ 5. Be as steady as you can.

CD: 5' in HRZ 1.

Day 6

WU: 15' in HRZ 1–2.

MS: Moderately long run in HRZ 2–3. Look to spend as much time in HRZ 3 as you can. This run should be no longer than 60–70 percent of your longest run in Phase 1.

CD: 5' in HRZ 1.

Day 7 Day OFF

WU:

MS:

CD:

PHASE 2 - WEEK 2

Day 1

WU: 10' in HRZ 1–2.

MS: 20–45' steady running in HRZ 2.

CD: 5' in HRZ 1.

***Day 2**

WU: 10' in HRZ 1–2.

MS: 20–45' steady running in HRZ 2.

CD: 5' in HRZ 1.

Day 3

WU: 15' in HRZ 1–3 + 4 × 30" building your speed to moderate fast by the end of each w/1' RI.

MS: 4–5 × 4' at SPZ 5 w/4' RI.

CD: 5' in HRZ 1.

***Day 4**

WU: 5' in HRZ 1.

MS: Short recovery run in HRZ 1–2. Or Day OFF.

CD: 5' in HRZ 1.

Day 5

WU: 10' in HRZ 1–2.

MS: 15–30' steady in SPZ 2.

CD: 5' in HRZ 1.

Day 6

WU: 30' in HRZ 1–3.

MS: 20–40' running on a hilly course between HRZ 3–5 based on the terrain. This should not be a long run, no longer than 60–70 percent of your longest run in Phase 1. Extend your run time in HRZ 2–3 to accomplish total run time goal for the day.

CD: 5' in HRZ 1.

Day 7 Day OFF

WU:

MS:

CD:

PHASE 2 - WEEK 3

Day 1

WU: 10' in HRZ 1–2.

MS: 20–45' steady running in HRZ 2.

CD: 5' in HRZ 1.

Day 2

WU: 15' in HRZ 1–3 + 4 × 30" building your speed to moderate fast by the end of each w/1' RI.

MS: 5–8 × 2' at SPZ 7 w/2' RI.

CD: 5' in HRZ 1.

***Day 3**

WU: 5' in HRZ 1.

MS: Short recovery run in HRZ 1–2. Or Day OFF.

CD: 5' in HRZ 1.

Day 4

WU: 15' in HRZ 1–3 + 4 × 30" building your speed to moderate fast by the end of each w/1' RI.

MS: 2–4 × 6–8' in HRZ 6 w/3' RI. Allow HR to build during the first minute or two—then hold steady.

CD: 5' in HRZ 1.

***Day 5**

WU: 10' in HRZ 1–2.

MS: 20–40' steady in SPZ 1.

CD: 5' in HRZ 1.

Day 6

WU: 30' in HRZ 1–3.

MS: 5 × 1' fast hill repeats w/2–3' RI. Run by what feels fast to you. Be consistent with each one. Then spend time in HRZ 2–5 on a hilly course before finishing with 5 × 1' fast hill repeats w/2–3' RI. This should not be a long run, no longer than 60–70 percent of your longest run in Phase 1.

CD: 5' in HRZ 1.

Day 7 Day OFF

WU:

MS:

CD:

PHASE 2 - WEEK 4

Day 1

WU: 10' in HRZ 1–2.

MS: 20–45' steady running in HRZ 2.

CD: 5' in HRZ 1.

Day 2 Day OFF

WU:

MS:

CD:

***Day 3**

WU: 10' in HRZ 1–2.

MS: 20–40' running in HRZ 2–3.

CD: 5' in HRZ 1.

Day 4

WU: 10' in HRZ 1–2.

MS: 20–40' steady in SPZ 1.

CD: 5' in HRZ 1.

Day 5 Day OFF

WU:

MS:

CD:

Day 6

WU: 30' in HRZ 1–3.

MS: 30–40' running on a hilly course between HRZ 3–5 based on the terrain. This should not be a long run, no longer than 50 percent of your longest run in Phase 1.

CD: 5' in HRZ 1.

Day 7 Day OFF

WU:

MS:

CD:

PHASE 2 - WEEK 5

Day 1

WU: 10' in HRZ 1–2.

MS: 20–45' steady running in SPZ 1.

CD: 5' in HRZ 1.

***Day 2**

WU: 10' in HRZ 1–2.

MS: 20–40' running in HRZ 2–3.

CD: 5' in HRZ 1.

Day 3

WU: 15' in HRZ 1–3 + 4 × 30" building your speed to moderate fast by the end of each w/1' RI.

MS: 4–6 × 3' at SPZ 6 w/3' RI.

CD: 5' in HRZ 1.

***Day 4**

WU: 5' in HRZ 1.

MS: Short recovery run in HRZ 1–2. Or Day OFF.

CD: 5' in HRZ 1.

Day 5

WU: 15' in HRZ 1–3 + 4 × 30" building your speed to moderate fast by the end of each w/1' RI.

MS: 20–40' in HRZ 5. Be as steady as you can.

CD: 5' in HRZ 1.

Day 6

WU: 20–30' in HRZ 1–3'.

MS: 20–40' running on a hilly course between HRZ 3–5 based on the terrain. This should not be a long run, no longer than 60–70 percent of your longest run in Phase 1. Extend your run time in HRZ 2–3 to accomplish total run time goal for the day.

CD: 5' in HRZ 1.

Day 7 Day OFF

WU:

MS:

CD:

PHASE 2 - WEEK 6

Day 1

WU: 10' in HRZ 1–2.

MS: 20–40' running in HRZ 2.

CD: 5' in HRZ 1.

Day 2

WU: 15' in HRZ 1–3 + 4 × 30" building your speed to moderate fast by the end of each w/1' RI.

MS: 5–6 × 4' at SPZ 5 w/4' RI.

CD: 5' in HRZ 1.

***Day 3**

WU: 5' in HRZ 1.

MS: Short recovery run in HRZ 1–2. Or Day OFF.

CD: 5' in HRZ 1.

Day 4

WU: 15' in HRZ 1–3 + 4 × 30" building your speed to moderate fast by the end of each w/1' RI.

MS: 10–20' steady running in HRZ 6.

CD: 5' in HRZ 1.

***Day 5**

WU: 5' in HRZ 1.

MS: Short recovery run in HRZ 1–2. Or Day OFF.

CD: 5' in HRZ 1.

Day 6

WU: 30' in HRZ 1–3.

MS: 40–60' of running on hilly course. On hills look to run in HRZ 4–6. On downhills and flat sections in HRZ 1–3. This should not be a long run, no longer than 60–70 percent of your longest run in Phase 1.

CD: 5' in HRZ 1.

Day 7 Day OFF

WU:

MS:

CD:

PHASE 2 - WEEK 7

***Day 1**

WU: 10' in HRZ 1–2.

MS: 20–40' running in HRZ 2.

CD: 5' in HRZ 1.

Day 2

WU: 15' in HRZ 1–3 + 4 × 30" building your speed to moderate fast by the end of each w/1' RI.

MS: 6–10 × 2' at SPZ 7 w/2' RI.

CD: 5' in HRZ 1.

***Day 3**

WU: 5' in HRZ 1.

MS: Short recovery run in HRZ 1–2. Or Day OFF.

CD: 5' in HRZ 1.

Day 4

WU: 15' in HRZ 1–3 + 4 × 30" building your speed to moderate fast by the end of each w/1' RI.

MS: 10–20' steady running in HRZ 6.

CD: 5' in HRZ 1.

Day 5

WU: 5' in HRZ 1.

MS: Short recovery run in HRZ 1–2.

CD: 5' in HRZ 1.

Day 6

WU: 30' in HRZ 1–3.

MS: 40–60' of running on hilly course. On hills look to run in HRZ 4–6. On downhills and flat sections in HRZ 1–3. This should not be a long run, no longer than 60–70 percent of your longest run in Phase 1.

CD: 5' in HRZ 1.

Day 7 Day OFF

WU:

MS:

CD:

PHASE 2 - WEEK 8

Day 1

WU: 5' in HRZ 1.

MS: Short recovery run in HRZ 1–2.

CD: 5' in HRZ 1.

Day 2 Day OFF

WU:

MS:

CD:

Day 3

WU: 10' in HRZ 1–2.

MS: 20–40' running in HRZ 2.

CD: 5' in HRZ 1.

Day 4

WU: 10' in HRZ 1–2.

MS: 20–40' Running in HRZ 2.

CD: 5' in HRZ 1.

Day 5 Day OFF

WU:

MS:

CD:

Day 6

WU: 30' in HRZ 1–3.

MS: 30–40' running on a hilly course between HRZ 3–5. Look to be as steady as you can in this zone regardless of the terrain. This should not be a long run, no longer than 50–60 percent of your longest run in Phase 1.

CD: 5' in HRZ 1.

Day 7 Day OFF

WU:

MS:

CD:

PHASE 2 - WEEK 9 OPTIONAL TEST WEEK

Day 1 Day OFF

WU:

MS:

CD:

Day 2

WU: 20–25' in HRZ 1–3 + 4 × 30" building your speed to moderate fast by the end of each w/1' RI.

TEST: At the track perform the same one-mile test that you did at the start of the program.

CD: 5' in HRZ 1.

***Day 3**

WU: 5' in HRZ 1.

MS: Short recovery run in HRZ 1–2.

CD: 5' in HRZ 1.

Day 4

WU: 10' in HRZ 1–2.

MS: 15–20' running in HRZ 2.

CD: 5' in HRZ 1.

Day 5

WU: 15' in HRZ 1–3 + 4 × 30" building your speed to moderate fast by the end of each w/1' RI.

TEST: At the track perform the 20-minute test and make training zone adjustments.

CD: 5' in HRZ 1.

Day 6

WU: 5–10' building to HRZ 2.

MS: HRZ 2–3 as you feel. Make this run 50 percent shorter than your longest run in Phase 1.

CD: 5' in HRZ 1.

Day 7 Day OFF

WU:

MS:

CD:

Self-guidance Tips

Remember, by working with your specific zones, the run program is individualized to your current state of fitness and ability. But it's quantum physics–hard to design a single schedule with times, intensities, distances, and workout frequencies for every runner out there, beginner to elite. Maybe you're just not ready to start out training six days a week. Maybe the 45-minute total run time on that first day is too short (if you're a veteran) or too long (if you're a beginner). Maybe you want to add days of training as you advance.

All of that is not only okay; it's essential. You have to listen to your body and be objective enough about your abilities to guide your own individual program. As you progress through the program, you'll see what you're capable of, and you'll settle into a daily and weekly run frequency and load that are right for you, based on your ability and the amount of time you have to train. As you work through the five-month program, your abilities will change. When they do, you can add more runs and make them longer.

Here are some tips on how to guide yourself throughout the program. Only you know your body and background; only you know what you need to do to realize your Cool Impossible. Embrace that, practice awareness, and execute accordingly.

1. Warm-up—As often as possible, integrate some run form awareness drills and slant board (or stability disk) sequence exercises into your prescribed warm-up in the foundation program. This will help activate your muscles and get them firing, and will also help you to remain consistent with foot strength training throughout the week. Do slant board one day and disk the next. You can do this before any run, but it should not replace your leg strength training for the day when you have the time.
2. Steady run—On the first day, I have you starting your steady run at a base of 20 to 45 minutes (for a total daily

running time with warm-up and cooldown of 35 to 60 minutes). If you're a beginner without much long-distance experience, you might feel better starting this steady run at 15 to 20 minutes (for a total run time of 30 to 35 minutes). If you're a veteran, you might want to start your steady run at 45 to 60 minutes (for a total run time of 60 to 75 minutes). But as you progress through the program, you might be able to handle longer times. Pay attention to your body, and adjust your efforts accordingly.

3. Managing intervals—On day three, there is a range given for the number of intervals to execute. Beginners should start on the lower end, and more experienced runners can jump to the higher number. Listen to your body and use your awareness.
4. Six days a week or not (the asterisk solution)—If you're an experienced runner, the idea of running six days a week is probably familiar to you. But if you're a beginner, you might turn to the first week of the schedule, see six days of runs with one day off, and go pale in the face. And the truth is that if you are a true beginner, you probably don't have the strength or endurance for that much running. So don't try to start there. Consider it a goal you're working toward. Start with three to four days a week. As you get stronger over time, increase your number of runs per week as you see fit. To help you adjust the training program to your personal needs, I've put asterisks next to suggested optional days that you could cut from the schedule. Once you're ready, just start adding these days back in. Whatever you do, stick closely to how I have laid out the weekly sequence and spacing of workouts and assigned intensities.
5. Rest intervals—Allow yourself enough rest to be able to perform your next interval run. Always use the re-

juvenation time, as it's as important as the work. When in doubt, err on the conservative side and take more rest. As a general rule, the more intense the run interval, the easier your rest interval should be. After more intense intervals, walk the entire rest interval or do an easy walk/run blend. After less intense intervals, run at a slow and easy pace, allowing your heart rate to drop to zone 1 or 2.

6. Breathing—When running easily, I suggest a pattern of one breath in and one out. As your effort increases to threshold level, I recommend going to a pattern of two breaths in and one breath out. At or near maximum effort, try two breaths in and two out. As always, experiment to see what works best for you.
7. Missing training days—My general rule for my athletes is, if you have to miss one or two days due to illness, life, or simply weather, skip it and move on with the schedule without making it up or adjusting the workouts. If you have to miss three to four days, or the week is completely interrupted, move the week of the program forward to the following week and continue with the program.
8. Trail runners—For those runners doing their longer, HR zone 2 to 3 workouts on trails, know that it will be difficult to maintain your HR in a steady zone on hilly terrain. You will find yourself working too hard on uphills and not hard enough on downhills. On these trail runs you can expand the HR zone range up to HR zone 5, which will keep you aerobic, but at this level you will not be training ideally for the purpose of these HR zone workouts. As best as you can, try to back off your effort on the hills during these runs or even power walk the hills. If you do most of your training on trails, I challenge you to get out on the road and do some flat

runs to help with your leg speed, economy, and aerobic endurance. During phase one, compromise a little by performing some of your long fat-burning workouts on roads and easy trails to get maximum benefit. Use your hilly trails for the workouts that call for higher HR zone intensity.

Heart-rate Self-measurement

With your nifty heart rate monitor, you'll be able to measure how your body is reacting to the workouts. Pay attention to these readings. It's awareness. Here are a few keys to watch for during the execution of the program:

- If your HR is lower than usual, and you feel like your effort is unusually high, this likely means your legs are tired and fatigued and need some R & R. Slow down or call it a day.
- If your HR is lower than usual, and even with increased effort you have a hard time elevating it, this likely means you're low on fuel. Eat something; see if it helps.
- Extreme heat will affect your HR and speed. Adjust your run accordingly. Slow down, lower intensity, or just realize your HR will be higher than normal and at a slower effort.
- Extreme cold will also affect your HR, likely lowering it by 5 to 7 beats versus your average. Do not force your effort to increase your HR. It is okay for it to be lower in cold temperatures.
- Every week, test your resting HR in the morning. First thing in the morning after waking, but before getting out of bed, monitor your HR for 2 to 5 minutes. The lower it is, the better. See if you find some improvement over the course of the training program.

FOUNDATION AWARENESS

All right, we're around Phelps Lake, and you've almost got everything you need to know about the strategic running foundation. I've walked you through the program; you're ready to roll.

Take one long last look at those crystal blue alpine waters. Then let's head back toward the trailhead. Wait, off to your left. See it through the trees? A black bear cub. Cute, right? Best we walk away, double time; mama bear can't be far behind—and good thing it isn't a grizzly cub. Your heart would really be racing then. . . . Keep on walking. I want to give you one more bit of parting advice.

When you're in the midst of the training program, I want you to be aware—mindful—of how your body is feeling, when your muscles and breathing effort are intense or relaxed, what it is like for you in each zone. Really be conscious of how your body is reacting every step of the way.

You might be one of those folks who really likes to let their mind wander as they run, to listen to music and just go away. That's fine—daydream; let yourself go free—but that does not mean that you can't still be mindful of how you are feeling. In fact, I would like you to discover that there is equal freedom in focusing your mind on your body, monitoring your breathing, heart rate, cadence, form, and the power left in your legs. This awareness is the true nature of athleticism. Practicing it will help you guide your own program, knowing when to push, when not to, how hard, how long, in your training. It will aid you in troubleshooting particular aches, pains, and levels of fatigue. When you get to races, this kind of awareness will pay dividends, because you'll be experienced in knowing how to set the proper pace and judging how much kick you have left in you near the finish line.

Finally, being aware throughout your training program will give you a level of confidence in—and knowledge of—your body, so that no ambition, no Cool Impossible will seem beyond your grasp. You'll know how good you are and how much better you can be.

6

EAT WELL, RUN WELL

COME JOIN ME for lunch at the Lotus Café, one of my favorites. It's pure mountain-town organic heaven, which, in a way, kind of sums up a lot of Jackson Hole.

You look well rested. Felt good to take the morning off, sleep late, and relax, right? Remember, how we treat our bodies while we're not training is just as important as how we do when we're training. Nowhere is that truer than when it comes to the food we eat. The old saying "Everything in moderation" is a classic, but in my opinion it leads only to being average. Being your best is a choice, and consistently making good nutrition choices leads to peak performance.

The Tarahumara Indians do nutrition right, and we can learn much from them. During my first day with the tribe of runners, when we set out on the thirty-mile trek toward Urique, the Tarahumara looked to be carrying no food, and they certainly had no hydration backpacks. On they marched, lean, tireless, up through the canyons, mile after mile. Halfway there or more, Manuel, who was leading us, stopped to take a rest. My fellow Americans and I had been munching on bars, sucking water through the tubes connected to our packs, and nibbling at any other stashes of food we'd brought. The Tarahumara had eaten nothing.

At one point, Manuel turned to us and smiled. Then, from under his loincloth, he produced a bag of pinole (ground toasted corn that makes for a nutrient-rich paste) and handmade corn tortillas. He was like a magician pulling a rabbit from a hat. Sitting on a ridge overlooking the canyon, he made a quick, simple energy snack—one rich in carbohydrates, and perfect support for the day's run. Everybody, including me, was discreetly watching his every bite.

Corn, beans, nuts, squash, chili peppers, wild greens, chia seeds, an occasional goat, chicken, or fish—these are the mainstays of the Tarahumara diet. They need nothing more to accomplish their incredible feats of endurance, and, I would argue, this diet contributes to their performance in a very real way.

But am I telling you to eat that way too? Not exactly. I consider their diet a good example, but by no means the rule of how I suggest we all need to eat.

Revolutionary, right? Not really. Eating well is pretty straightforward. For centuries, the Tarahumara have been eating a simple, non-diverse diet in Copper Canyon, one low in sugar and cholesterol, and high in fiber, complex carbohydrates, vitamins, and other nutrients.

And as far as the diversity of their diet goes, we might all be better off living in a canyon, far from civilization, where we can eat only what we forage and grow ourselves. Instead, we live in a society with a vast array of food, most of it overprocessed, oversugared, oversize junk.

Was that me banging the table with my fist?

Listen, we have a choice of how we want to eat. We know what is best for us: simple, natural, nutrient-dense foods. The challenge is choosing to eat that way, making it a habit, and sticking with that choice. It takes discipline, focus, awareness.

Not to sound like a drill sergeant, but too many people say they want to be fit, healthy, thin, toned, and low in body fat, but they're unwilling to do what's necessary to make that happen. Your actions need to match your goal. In your training, you cannot expect to run a sub-three-hour marathon by training twenty miles a week. The same equation works with nutritional health; consistency reaps the highest benefits. Keep your pace steady in eating the right foods, and I guarantee you the benefits will be profound. You'll have more energy, more lean muscle, more vibrant skin, better performance, and a better quality of health and life.

It's not discipline for its own sake. Practicing discipline makes us feel good about ourselves, and this empowers us further. Ironically, it is the pleasures and comforts we're scared to lose that ultimately lead to unhappiness.

So take a look at that Lotus Café menu. See what strikes you as something the Tarahumara might eat. Over the day, I'll give you a little minicourse on how to fuel your body, from everyday nutrition to what you need for training and races.

One final word before our waitress comes over and takes our order: I will not give you any hard-and-fast rules. That's not my place, and I don't think it's effective. A lot of this is mental, a conscious decision you have to make. You have a choice as to how you want to eat, how far you want to dedicate yourself to improving your diet, same as you do with your training. The better you eat, the better you will feel and perform as a runner. Nutrition has a cumulative effect, just like good form and fitness.

I'll give you a road map to reach what I consider the ideal and allow you the opportunity to choose how far you want to push yourself to reach it. That's my job as your coach.

EVERYDAY NUTRITION

I am not a doctor, and I don't have an advanced degree in nutrition. My understanding of how and what we should eat to improve our performance as runners and better our lives comes from classroom study, clinical collaborations at universities, my own self-directed studies, personal experience, and lessons drawn from my athletes. What I've learned from those sources is that we will all feel and do better from the same basic diet. Yes, there are people with health concerns who require special dietary decisions and alterations, but just as with physical training, I feel the majority of us are similar and respond to simple, nutrient-rich eating. I think what you'll find here makes a lot of simple common sense.

Take a look at what I ordered at Lotus. We've been together for a few days, so you're probably not surprised to see a salad again, this time my favorite: steamed brown basmati coconut rice, sautéed broccoli, red pepper, zucchini, red onion, spinach, and carrot—all topped with fresh mango and a little buffalo meat. I'm not counting calories or divvying up my meal by grams of carbs, fats, and proteins. It's more of an eyeballing, a general sense of things.

And here's the general sense: First, I want lots of organic fruits and vegetables; the sky's the limit, really, for these kinds of carbohydrates. Carbs, along with fat, provide us with our main source of energy, whether we use it immediately or later. They do some good work for the function of our muscles, kidneys, brain, and nervous system, and, when rich in fiber, they're aces for our digestive tract too. Yeah, carbs! So just forget all those diets that tell you to avoid carbs. Just be sure you're getting them from fruits and veggies and not from refined or processed foods. You want the kind of carbs that come in natural, nutrient-rich foods. We need those vitamins and all that other good stuff that comes from plant-based food.

What does that mean? Well, if you have a burrito, do an open-faced burrito, or lose the wrap entirely. All that pasta—that's processed wheat, and not so great. Same with white bread; stick to the whole-grain kinds, or even better yet, skip all breads. Just remember, you don't want a no-carb diet; you want a right-carb diet.

Second, let's talk about protein. In all my meals, I typically eat some kind of plant-based protein or lean meat or fish. But I usually have a portion that is no bigger than the palm of my hand. That lean buffalo on my favorite Lotus salad roughly achieves that size.

Protein grows and heals tissue. Protein provides the building blocks of muscle, and if you're doing my training program, you're building that in all the right places. Best as I can, I stick with organic, free-range meats and wild-caught fish. Again, aim for the natural, like the Tarahumara (though I can't vouch for their fishing techniques, which on occasion include throwing explosives into bodies of water to stun the fish so they can grab them when they float to the surface).

Finally, let's talk about fat. You'll notice I'm not having avocados today. I love my avocados and nuts. But the buffalo meat has fat, and the veggies were likely sautéed in oil, and even if not, there's the coconut and yummy grapeseed-oil salad dressing. So my meal is far from fat-free (and that's a good thing). Overall, fat gets a bad rap. It's essential for absorbing vitamins and protecting our major organs, and it's also a source of energy and gives us a full, satisfied feeling. So keep in mind that fat is a necessary nutrient, but you have to eat the right kind of fat. The more natural the source—nuts, avocados—the better. But you can't have too much of it. Pay attention to how much fat is in your meal, so you know when you need more—and when you don't. My salad here at the Lotus has just the right amount of good fat in it, so I don't add any avocado or nuts.

For those of you who like numbers rather than the idea of eyeballing the right proportions, I'll give you a factoid. Studies show that the diet of the Tarahumara breaks down in the following way: 80 percent carbs, 10 percent protein, and 10 percent fat. Don't get too caught up in this formula, though, nor in calorie counts or the latest trends, like vegan, veggie or paleo. For me—and I know this is a personal choice—those kinds of labels inhibit my ability to learn and be open, to experiment and see how different foods make me feel. Some days I eat like a vegetarian; other days I have meat and eggs.

Instead of carbs, fats, proteins, calorie counts, or food fads, I want to stress the quality of the foods you are eating. We know we need fuel for our bodies, but to use the well-worn analogy of a car, the kind of fuel we're pumping into our tanks is critical to our performance. We constantly regenerate cells within our body, and this means everything we put into our mouth affects every part of us. Think about that for a minute. You can put an extremely low-grade gasoline into your car. The tank will take it. The car will move, but it'll be sluggish, and over time it'll break down more quickly, sure as there's a side of the road. But if you use a high-octane gasoline, you'll hear that engine hum, and off you go. Zoom.

You have to decide that you're willing to make the effort to keep putting the best fuel at hand into the tank. Initially, this effort may feel like a sacrifice and a chore. But the better you eat, the better you'll feel both physically and mentally, and the more you will crave good food. Your good choices will create a cycle that makes your effort to eat well easier and, soon enough, one you like and enjoy.

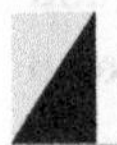

Eric's No-recipe Daily Diet

For more guidance on how to eat naturally, simply, here's a day in my life at the table. Use what you want from what I do, but be forewarned that I'm not big on following or giving rigid recipes. I prefer to have a bunch of fresh staples in the house—some chopped veggies at the ready, spices on hand—and just wing it. As I'm the cook at home, this helps me keep it simple and uncomplicated—two key factors that allow me to be consistent and true to a more natural diet. I primarily look at food as fuel, and this drives my daily food choices.

Breakfast—The first thing I do is hit a double espresso. This gets the fire going and is part of my morning ritual, relaxing sitting on the deck staring at the mountains, daydreaming and visualizing an aspect of my Cool Impossible and planning my run for the day. I usually wait a couple hours after getting out of bed to eat my first meal. For me, it's a form of fasting, which makes me alert. Once I do have breakfast, it's usually a couple of fried eggs over a corn tortilla with an avocado on top. On the side, I'll have a banana or cantaloupe. Other days, it'll be an omelet with a bunch of stuff thrown inside (spinach, kale, tomatoes), or a smoothie with frozen fruit, cashews, and chia seeds.

Lunch—Leftovers. I love leftovers, particularly for lunch. It makes life easy and the meal quick. Usually I'll have some salmon or buffalo steak from the night before. I'll get a bowl, mix in some avocado and olive oil, toss in some fresh spinach, and have a salad. Or I might take the same and fold it into a corn tortilla spread with hummus for my own style of taco. On the side, I have more fruit.

Prerun Snack—If I run in the morning, I use breakfast for fuel. When I'm taking a long run, I'll add some sweet potatoes to my omelet and fruit, or a side of oatmeal, depending on the length and demand of the run. For short runs, the smoothie will do. If I want to hit the trails in the early afternoon, I time the run an hour or so after lunch, so that my meal serves as prerun fuel. If it's later, I'll have a snack thirty or forty minutes before, typically a slice of whole-wheat bread with almond butter and chia seeds, or that yummy chia smoothie again.

Dinner—At home or out to eat, I'm a big fan, as you undoubtedly know, of salads. I love spinach and kale especially. They pack a huge punch of nutrients. When I'm making my own salad, my favorite is seared tuna with spinach and heaps of raw veggies: red peppers, cucumbers, and tomatoes. Throw in a little sea salt, an avocado, and some olive oil, and you have a meal. I also like salmon with sweet potatoes and asparagus.

Snacks—I'm not a big snacker other than what is needed for exercise. If I'm hungry, I make a meal or, at the least, a smoothie.

Water and Herbal Tea—You won't find me with soda and rarely with a sports drink. Short of my espresso in the morning, I drink water all day. At night, I'll make a mug of herbal tea and relax.

THE DEMON IN THE AISLES

At the start, getting into this cycle of good food choices will not be easy. Let's address why, but before that, finish up your lunch. Then come with me. We'll take a quick drive across Jackson to the big-box grocery store. Its name is irrelevant. Most of them are the same, and I'm sure this is one is no different from the one in your hometown.

We enter through the automatic doors. After all, why should we be bothered to use our bodies to open a door? We're looking for convenience here, and if there's one thing about grocery stores, they make bad choices very convenient. Walk around with me. Notice how the whole foods—the fresh fruit and vegetables, the fresh-butchered meat and newly caught fish—are all located around the periphery of the store. In terms of the square footage of the rest of the big-box, they take up almost no space. Meanwhile, in the heart of the store, in aisle after aisle, row after row, are shelves stacked high with processed, preserved, and industrially manufactured "food."

Follow me to the cereal section. Take a look at the cartoon-character-festooned boxes. Look at their nutrition labels. And then look farther down the aisle at the cereals packaged as "nutritious and healthy." In both you'll see there are grams and grams of what I consider to be the biggest, most pervasive, most insidious drug in this country today: sugar. In my opinion—and there are quite a few experts backing me up—it's an addiction problem for many of us that is no different from alcohol or cigarettes, with similar cravings and equally devastating effects. High levels of fructose, corn syrup, and sucrose (whether beet or sugarcane) in our food and drink are part of the problem.

Sugar in high amounts is everywhere in this store, from cereals to breads, pastas, sauces, juices, snacks, ready-made meals, and on and on. You'd be surprised at where you'll find the demon lurking. Getting a yogurt? Check the label and be prepared to be wowed. Instant oatmeal? Yep, there too. Even the packaged bagels have it.

These types of sugar-steeped foods are bad for you in three ways.

One, the amount of sugar is difficult for your body to process. Some argue, particularly in terms of high fructose, that it is plain toxic for your body. Two, these foods serve up empty, nutrient-stripped calories. You fill up on sugar and don't have the room or appetite for foods with the vitamins, minerals, and antioxidants that would be much better for your body. Three, these foods are addictive and cause overeating. The more sugar you eat, the more you crave.

If you're eating a lot of processed foods, you may not know you have a sugar problem, but even if you're not a sweet-and-treat addict, it's likely you do. I did. Sugar is hiding in so many processed foods, it's not just a question of eating too many candy bars and cookies. So let's do something about it as the first step in reshaping our everyday eating.

Come on. I need to grab a cart and do some shopping while I tell you what's ahead. If some clerks or stackers wave hello, don't be surprised. I come here two or three times a week. It helps me plan meals and keep fresh, natural food in the house, and the processed box stuff out—most of all, the sugary stuff.

THE TWENTY-DAY SUGAR DETOX

As an athlete and coach, I'm always looking for an edge, trying new things, seeing what works, what doesn't, to boost performance and raise my game to the next level. When I first moved to Jackson Hole, I found myself away from my usual routine, so I decided to go to the extreme to get a true sense of the rewards that eating well can give us. As a coach, I like to use myself as a guinea pig to see what kinds of things bring improved performance. So, as an experiment, I focused on cutting out sugar from my diet. Save for sugar in fruits, I'm talking a complete ban. Keep in mind that up to this point, I had a pretty good diet already. It wasn't like I wolfed down sweets all day. But I had never focused on the hidden sugars that find their way into our foods, and I decided now to hunt them out and get rid of them.

The cravings came and went; sometimes the impulse to grab some granola and yogurt was tough to resist. But if I was aware of them and could wait them out, impulses like that would always pass. You just have to give them time. After a few weeks, the cravings went away. (I've heard some people say it took only a few days for the cravings to stop when they cut out all sugar.) Meanwhile, I dropped five pounds. I had already been lean, but now I was even leaner. But I didn't feel starved. I felt more sated at meals, yet less full. I had more energy. In terms of performance, after three weeks of my sugar detox, I was able to run to the top of Snow King five minutes faster at the same level of effort. In a word, I was amazed. There was a very dramatic improvement in my overall athletic performance. In a very short period, my body transformed in a way that it would have taken months of training to achieve.

Convinced? If you want to enjoy these benefits yourself, here is your challenge: a twenty-day sugar detox. Now, a good time to do this detox is during the transition/rejuvenation phase of your run program, when your energy needs will be at their lowest, but if you're supermotivated to begin straightaway, you can do that too. Your goal here is simple: no sugar except from fruits. Check the labels of everything you eat. Under carbohydrates, there should be a line for sugar. You want that to be zero. As for the rest of your diet, it should remain the same.

Why this extreme move? You will lose the weight, but that's not it, even though for some of us, shedding a quick five to ten pounds is a pretty nice side benefit. Foremost, I want to make you aware of what you eat and how it affects you physically and mentally. Consider this the foundation for moving forward.

As in setting any good foundation, there's some tough work ahead. This detox will not be easy. Many of you likely believe you don't consume much sugar. Take this on; try it and see. As well as we think we're eating, it's hard to do away with this little invader, and you'll be surprised at how much sugar ends up in your daily eating habits. In the first week, you will likely crave it in its absence and, in many respects, find it simply hard to create meals without sugar. You might get cranky, lethargic, antsy, or all three in the space of a short time. Sounds great, right?

Here are some tips on how to get through it: Drink lots of water and be prepared with healthy snacks like celery, carrots, nuts, and dried fruit to munch on. Eat a lot of salads. Hit the juice bar or make your own (but with only fresh fruits and veggies—nothing processed!), and avoid any yogurt with sugar in it. Weigh yourself frequently; start creating some awareness of how fueling affects weight and impacts how you feel. Enroll your family or friends (or both!) to keep you motivated and on track. Eat simple and repetitive meals; they will help you organize and stick to the detox.

After a week, things will get easier. The cravings will pass. After two weeks, you will likely start to radiate health and find yourself more energetic and focused than ever. Enjoy it.

Good or bad feelings, ill or revved up, be aware of your body and your thoughts about food throughout this process. This awareness is fundamental. Be aware of what you eat, and how the sustained absence of sugar makes you feel. It's the key to your success in finishing your detox—and the chief reason you're doing it.

MODERATION IS MEDIOCRITY—95/5

We're here at the big-box grocery store so you can see what types of food you'll need to bring into your house to eat healthfully. I practice what I preach—and I don't like to do things halfway. But let me be clear: When I use the word moderation in terms of your diet, I am not talking portion control. If you're eating well, and paying attention to when you feel full, this is not really an issue. Instead, I am focused on your overall food choices.

Check out my shopping cart. Watch what I grab as we walk around the store. And I mean around the periphery, where they typically keep the fresh stuff. We won't be taking too many dives into the middle.

There's too much temptation and hidden sugar in those aisles.

While I hit the produce section, heaping lots of fruits and vegetables into my cart—spinach, kale, apples, bananas, cabbage, cantaloupe, broccoli, sweet potatoes, avocados, red peppers, squash, any seasonal ripe fruits—let's project ahead once your twenty days of detox are over.

At that point, I want you to sit down and think again about how you feel. You have done something pretty extreme. But my bet is, you feel terrific. You've lost weight. You spring out of bed; you're not as tired at night. Your skin looks fresh. More than the physical, I also wager you're feeling pretty darn proud of yourself. You did a hard thing: You succeeded in sticking to the plan and freeing yourself from sugar. You've started to create a new philosophy of how you want to eat, and you've stuck to it. That perseverance, that discipline makes you feel good about yourself and your choices.

Consider, then, what it would be like if you had just given up a little sugar in your diet. Maybe you committed to a breakfast detox or dinner detox instead of an all-day detox. Do you think you'd feel better? Maybe a little, but the change would be less noticeable. As a result, you'd be less convinced that you're on the right path. That's why I say moderation is mediocrity. If we don't shoot for the stars, we won't even get off the ground.

And the truth is that it's likely that no matter how diligent you were during the detox, you eliminated at most only 95 percent of the sugar in your diet. Don't be discouraged. I think a 95 percent simple, natural diet, and a 5 percent do-whatever-you-want-go-crazy diet, is a spectacular way to live. If you eat well 95 percent of the time, you're shooting for the stars. I'm not a monk who forbids all earthly pleasures. I like my cold Newcastle beers and my chocolate-chip cookies. But I limit them to only 5 percent of my diet. That doesn't mean I consume them "in moderation." It means I practically avoid them completely. That's enough to make a real difference in how you feel, a convincing difference.

Again, my aim is for you to feel how good it is possible to feel. At 95/5, you'll know.

THE TWENTY-DAY WHOLE-FOOD CHALLENGE

We're almost through the grocery store. I've got what I need for the next few days: A bag of fifty corn tortillas—no fillers. Some fresh ahi tuna and wild-caught salmon. We had some fun at the butcher counter, right? I love the local game here. The lean elk meat will grill up nicely. We loaded up on eggs, frozen raspberries and blueberries for smoothies (remember: no added sugar), and we got some almonds and cashews from the bulk bins. We dived briefly into the middle aisles for some olive oil, beans, and cans of tomatoes.

I almost forgot—we need to hit the spices. Got to rev up the taste. Some thyme, basil, rosemary, chili. Oh, while we're here, grab some salsa; it's got lots of flavor and, with the right brand, no sugar.

As we check out and load up my truck, let's talk about your second challenge. Hopefully this shopping excursion has given you some inspiration.

Once you've detoxed from sugar, I want you to focus on eating as simply and naturally as possible. Keep up your 95/5 ratio for sugar, and now let's shoot for the same extreme end of eating well: no junk food, no processed foods, no bread, no pasta, no cheese, no yogurt, no alcohol, no cereal, no granola. Did you see any of those in my cart? And cow's milk—you can do without that too. Fruits and vegetables, as well as kidney and black beans, are loaded with the calcium you need.

Eat only simple, whole foods. When you're shopping back home, remember this little trip. If you need more help deciding whether you should be eating something, imagine you're living on a farm a couple hundred years ago. You pick the location. Eat only what would be available then: what the farmer and his family could keep as livestock, grow in their fields, hunt in the forest, or fish in the lakes. It's that simple. Avoid the processed foods of our modern society. Eat food that remembers where it came from, foods without ingredient lists, or with simple ones that don't include any words you can't pronounce. Eat real food.

Over the course of this second challenge, I'm also going to urge you to raise the bar on your awareness of how the food you put in your mouth makes you feel. In particular:

1. Notice the difference between being hungry and wanting something to eat.
2. Notice how little you need to eat to feel full and satisfied when your diet is made up of only real, whole foods.
3. Notice how balanced and stable your energy is when you have a balanced meal of carbs/fat/protein.
4. Notice how your body, skin, and muscles feel in the morning when you incorporate fruit with your breakfast.
5. Notice how your weight changes. Some say don't use a scale while reworking your diet. I say baloney. See how meals and various diet changes work themselves out in your weight on a daily basis.
6. Notice how feeling good from eating drives you to want this feeling all the time.
7. Finally, notice what happens those times when you go for the pizza or ice cream. Ask yourself whether the pleasure you get from eating it—and the bad feeling afterward—is better than the great feeling you get when you choose not to eat the pizza or ice cream at all.

Once you've finished these two twenty-day challenges, I promise you'll understand, perhaps better than at any other time in your life, how what we eat affects who we are, both physically and mentally. Now you're ready to define for yourself what everyday nutritional health means to you.

NUTRITION MISSION STATEMENT

After all this talk of what to eat and what not to eat, you've earned yourself a home-cooked meal. Come back to my house. We'll sit out back, take in the cloudless afternoon sky, crank the Alarm on the speakers, and write down your goals for eating. Then later, maybe after a walk down to the creek, I'll cook for you.

As your coach, I want you to reach for the best that's in you. I want you to realize your Cool Impossible as a runner and as a person. Therefore, I urge you to shoot for the ideal in terms of eating; always choose the healthiest course, no matter the discipline required and the temptations resisted. If you do, I promise you will feel so good. You'll fall in love with the new you. And you'll be empowered to continue eating well and living your life as your best self.

My diet is a choice, and I'm happy with it. I choose to eat simply and naturally at most every meal. If I decide to go for those cookies, first and foremost it is a conscious choice. I have the treat and I enjoy it, but I also decide to go without the same for several weeks. I shoot for the 95/5 because I like how it makes me feel. In a way, I make it almost a game to see how well I can live, how long I can live, knowing I'm eating the best I can. Plus, it gives me a heck of a base for my own running.

But my life is not yours. You have to make your own nutritional choices. That said, be clear about your goals. Have a plan and an awareness to eat well. Have a nutrition mission statement and use it as your guide and inspiration. Let's try to put one together now, but I also urge you to review, rethink, and rephrase it once you finish your own two challenges.

Your nutritional ambitions should match your running ambitions. The better you want to be at running, the better you should eat. If you want to perform athletically at the highest level for you, then you will have to commit to a nutrition-rich, junk-free diet. We're talking 95/5 here. Put it in the statement.

Or you might want to set times to be more or less rigorous with your diet. Maybe you'll choose a time on the calendar when you want to be at your best—and therefore eat the best. This could be a three- to five-month period. In your statement, dedicate to beginning this transition a month before the period; then execute for the three to five months at 95/5; then back off afterward, just as you handle the training around a big race.

Or you might want to start your nutritional transformation more gradually after your two challenges, then gather steam month-to-month for a full-out 95/5 commitment.

The mission statement is up to you. Make a choice based on your goals. Do what is good for you, stick to it, and you'll *want* to stick to it.

STRATEGIC FUELING

We've spent the day together. We've examined general nutrition—what's best to eat and why. We've had two meals, written down a mission statement. I've cooked for you, no less. And yet, I'm betting you're a little dissatisfied. All this time, we've only briefly touched on what to eat before and during our runs and races.

Relax; have some green tea. Let's sit down out back and tone things down with a little Jeff Buckley for your ears. Check out that sky. Have you imagined so many stars were possible?

By getting your everyday eating on the right path, you are working on what you need to do to train and race. By building the foundation and putting emphasis on your daily eating habits, you'll reap much greater returns than with some secret meal you have before or after a specific run. It's no less important than working on your strength, form, and training schedule. To finish an ultramarathon, you won't succeed by skimping on your day-to-day miles. Same goes for skimping on the right kind of food in the weeks and months before a race.

After coaching many runners and athletes, I've learned that proper fueling on training and race days is a fickle beast. What works perfectly for one athlete fails with another. What works great for one athlete one race might not work for this same athlete in the next. On any given day, there are so many factors at play. Sometimes you're feeling it, sometimes not. In cycling, we often refer to this simply as having a "bad legs day" or a "good legs day." It's important to learn from each, to see what works and what doesn't.

There are three things I know for sure: One, building the right foundation is critical. We've covered that. Two, being fueled before a run or race keeps that body moving. Three, being fit aids your fuel efficiency, allowing you to get more out of what you eat.

Prerun Fueling

Knowing what to eat before a training run depends on how long you'll be running and at what intensity, as well as when you last ate. Take a step back, though, and the whole trick is awareness. You have to pair the amount of fuel you need to the type of exercise you're doing. With a little common sense and planning, you'll be in good shape.

Here I'll break down some different, but very typical runs during your training week to give you the broad strokes of what you should be eating beforehand:

1. Short, easy run (HR zone 1 to 3): These runs usually come during the workweek for me, and I won't need much, if any, fueling beforehand other than the meals I'm normally eating that day.
2. Short, fast run or interval training (HR zone 4 to 7, SP zone 3 to 7): Thirty to forty-five minutes before this run, have something on the light side, like a smoothie with fruit and chia, or a couple handfuls of cashews and fruit.
3. Long run (HR zone 1 to 3): These runs are low to moderate in tempo, but they are your longest effort. For most of us, these are weekend runs. Keep in mind that a good solid meal the night before helps. Then, one to two

hours before the run, fuel up well, based on the exact distance planned. (I like eggs and/or oatmeal with fruit and nuts on top in the morning if I'm heading out for a few hours on the trail.)

Like I said, these are very broad strokes of advice and by no means ironclad rules. If you want to get it right, you have to be mindful of when you last ate and what fuel demands you will make on your body during your run. Say you're heading out the office door at two p.m. for an hour run, but because the phone was ringing off the hook, you haven't eaten since breakfast. Well, you might think about eating something before that easy run.

The true insight—and fun—comes with awareness, testing to see what exactly you need to eat or drink to reach your highest level of performance, both before a run and during it. Be aware, and try different things; see what works for you. Learn what works for you on different days, based on the different ways you can feel because of how much you slept that night or how much stress you have at work right now. Eat more or fewer carbs or proteins at your prerun meal. Eat a half hour, versus two hours, before you hit the trail. Try different strategies until you find the right ones for you.

Things won't go right all the time, but that's kind of the point. We learn from our failures, and usually we learn a lot more from them than from our successes. When experimenting, feel your level of energy during different parts of your run. All other things being equal (e.g., terrain, temperature), when do you feel at your best or worst during the run? Also, keep weighing yourself before and after runs. Note the demands your running is making on your body. Are you gaining or losing weight? Are you staying the same? Getting on that scale is an awareness tool, allowing you to understand how your nutrition and training are affecting your body.

Over time, practicing awareness, you should get a sense of your overall level of fitness and the impact your fueling has in a "good legs" or "bad legs" day.

In the Thick of It—Midrun Fueling Advice

When you're running long distances, it's important to know how to fuel on the go. But here as elsewhere, everyone is different. You have to experiment and understand what works best for you during training runs and races, and be prepared to troubleshoot while out there. There are so many things available—gels, beans, sports drinks, bars, trail mix, dried fruit, and honey. I know. I know: Most of these are high in sugar and not so natural, but particularly with races, convenience wins out. Anyway, you're burning that simple sugar pretty quick.

There are no hard-and-fast rules for when and how much fuel to take. It depends on what distance and amount of time you're running, terrain, intensity, and temperature. Especially when it comes to hydration and fueling, I feel like many people rely on strict rules that can sometimes get them in trouble.

Here's quick insight into what I do. Use the following as a stepping-off point for your own experimentation. Typically, I organize my fueling based on time running, rather than distance:

Thirty to Seventy-five Minutes

Given that I'm on track with my own 95/5 nutrition mission statement, and I've followed my prerun fueling practice, I will not fuel during these runs. As for water, unless it's superhot, I drink only when thirsty, rather than following any kind of strict regimen about hydration.

Seventy-five Minutes to Two Hours

This time segment can sometimes be the most challenging to figure out. On easy runs of this distance, you might not need much fuel, relying on your prerun strategy. But I will always take something with me on these easy runs, most times an oat-based energy bar, just in case I need it. Usually when I need fuel on easy runs, it is due more to the cumulative training load of my week rather than the specific demands of the run itself. Practice awareness; ask yourself how demanding the last few days have been, as this might determine whether you need more fuel during an easy effort at this distance. I take water, and drink to quench my thirst.

When training at a quick pace or racing in this time frame, I will tap into my 5 percent allotment and use gels about seventy-five to ninety minutes into the run if I feel my reserves are depleted and an energy pickup could do me some good. Again, this is for convenience and function (and it's hard to digest "real" food during high-intensity running). The key is that you don't need much, just a little something in your system to finish out the run. When using gels, I will drink water more consistently.

Two to Five Hours

On trails, and when the intensity fluctuates from easy to moderate, I try to stick to real foods and water. I look for natural oat-type bars, dates, or dried fruit with nuts. At an hour and a half to two hours into a run, I will begin to fuel, spacing the fueling times out by forty-five to sixty minutes for the duration of the run.

If the run is long but easy and fat-burning, I might focus on a big meal an hour before the run and then see how far I can go before I need fuel, then fuel once I need it and continue to fuel as needed. This is the time you learn what your body needs and how it responds to fuel.

For water, if it's an average-temperature day, I like to make sure I'm getting roughly twenty-four ounces every seventy-five to ninety minutes, and will then be sure to hydrate after the run. You do not need to go over-the-top with hydration. Just be as consistent as you can and do your best with what you can carry. I use handheld bottles and hydration packs when needed.

During a race, when it's a fast, sustained effort, I rely on the convenience of gels or honey. I fuel more frequently, understanding that the higher demands of the distance at high intensity will burn carbohydrates faster. In races, I typically use water for hydration, using sports drinks only occasionally as a change of pace, because I'm already taking gels and don't need the double dose of sugar. I've found consuming sports drinks and gels together causes stomach issues, so it's best to rely mostly on water for hydration. Find what works for you, and be sure to drink water with your gels.

Five Hours and Beyond

The single most important thing about fueling during long, long runs and races is to eat and drink when you feel good, because when you don't feel good, the last thing you'll want to do is eat or drink. Think ahead; act accordingly.

Otherwise, I maintain the same fuel and water timing periods as in the two-to-five-hour run, albeit with some added awareness. When the intensity is lower, I eat energy bars and "real" food. As the intensity heightens, I switch to gels. If my heart rate seems to dip low and I lose alertness, I know it is a sign to eat. I also evaluate my effort levels each hour by looking at the course demands and my heart rate. Some sections are more demanding than others, and therefore you need to adjust your fueling during and after these accordingly.

This is very important and will help prevent stomach issues: If you are running an easier stretch and know a long hill or tougher section is coming, start fueling when your stomach can deal better with the intake. When intensity heightens, your stomach has a harder time digesting fuel, so back off on eating for a while. Just be sure to fuel again after this tough section, when the intensity lowers. By practicing awareness and avoiding a strict fueling regimen, you'll avoid a lot of stomach issues.

In training and running ultras, listen to your cravings and experiment. At these long distances, the only rule is to do what really works for you based on what you have learned in practice. Some racers love bacon, finding the fat really helps them midrace. So when training it's important to try different fueling strategies. On some long runs, fuel frequently (but with smaller portions). On others, fuel less frequently (but with bigger portions). Through these experiments, learn as much as you can about your body, what it needs, what it likes at certain times throughout the run, day or night. The key is awareness: How is your stomach feeling; how has your water intake been the last hour; how were your intensity-effort demands the last hour; what do you have up ahead; is there a big climb? Questions like this are meant to give you a reading on your own body, like a fuel gauge tells you how much gas is left in your car. These questions help you figure out when and how much fuel you'll need on the road ahead.

NUTRITION AND YOUR COOL IMPOSSIBLE

Time to call it a night. Go back to your hotel; work on that nutrition mission statement a little more. Before you go to sleep, I want you to mull over our talk today. There were lots of specifics: carbs, sugar, twenty-day detoxes, and what exactly makes for the kind of diet that will allow you to excel.

But there was much more. Throughout our runs and chats over the past few days, I've spoken again and again about awareness. I don't know whether you noticed, but today I talked about it more than ever. Being aware of what you put in your body, how it makes you feel, is super important. Yet this comes second to the awareness you need of your ambitions as a runner. Only with a clear awareness of your overall goals can you make the necessary commitment to the kind of healthy diet you need to achieve them.

The Cool Impossible demands an understanding of the type of runner you want to be, the conviction that you can do it, and a willingness to put in the effort to make it happen. In reshaping your nutritional habits, you'll learn to love what I call "digging the dirt." At first, you might find it an effort to stick to your two twenty-day challenges. But if you're aware, and you continue on the course you set, you'll realize how good you feel—not only physically, but also for taking hold of a new philosophy of living and being. Your discipline becomes its own satisfaction, and your success at maintaining it will give you confidence and a sense of empowerment to continue.

In some ways, eating well is like digging for gold. We dig, dig, dig, keeping to the effort, until one day we find a nugget. The find makes us happy, but we soon realize we've also fallen in love with the effort of digging. Awareness leads us to this understanding, and there is so much more it can do if we know how to tap into its power.

7

PUTTING IT ALL TOGETHER

LOTS TO DO today, a long run/hike, so let's start the day right and get a good breakfast. We get together early—yes, that sun just rose over the mountains—to talk at the Bunnery. Smell those eggs and that fresh coffee brewing. The locals love this diner, and for good reason.

Grab a seat. We won't be here too long, but I know you've had some questions about how to piece together the strength, form, foundation, and nutrition programs. Let's cover that before we head off today to dive into the big kahuna: awareness and realizing your Cool Impossible.

THE BASIC QUESTIONS

So you want to know when you should start? The answer is, as soon as you return home and get the equipment you need. In other words, as soon as you can, go straight into strength training. Begin getting those feet, legs, and upper body good and strong. As you're building strength, it's a great time to begin your performance running transition program. Buy those zero-drop shoes and slowly work up your miles in them. As I've said before, strength helps form; form helps strength. This is also the perfect time to begin changing how you eat. Launch into your first twenty-day challenge. In sum, the first three to six weeks of your training are really your athletic transition time to let your body adapt to strength, form, new shoes, and nutrition. In a perfect world, this is the ideal way to start.

During this time, don't worry about how you should integrate the strength training with run form work on a day-to-day basis. Forget about a specific schedule of workouts for different days of the week right now. This is a time of limited running. You have more opportunity here to dive into the strength. Optimally, you're working strength five to six days a week, alternating lower body and upper body. Run on the same days you're doing the lower-body strength work, preferably running first. In this period, you really want to get a feel for how your body is responding, where you're sore, where you're not.

Some people ask me once they're finished with the run transition program, do they really need the preparation phase before they leap into the meat of the program? Quick answer: yes. Long answer: The preparation phase is just that, meant to prepare the legs and cardiovascular system with consistency and endurance so your body is primed for the start of the foundation program. During the preparation phase, continue strength training, continue your nutrition work with your second twenty-day challenge, and continue your form awareness and drills. Use this time to put yourself in the best place possible to begin the foundation program.

So, once you're in the five-month foundation program, you might wonder whether you should stop doing my strength training. People ask me that a lot. But remember: I've said you can never stop getting better. That means you should continue with your strength training. The good news is that your body has already adapted to the new demands you're making on it, and you will reap further performance gains and build athleticism. Follow the lower-body/upper-body sequencing schedule that I suggested in chapter three, so that you're allowing your body proper recovery time. In addition, you also want to continue with your awareness of form. At this time as well, you should begin developing and executing your nutrition mission statement.

SELF-COACHING

Now, take a minute, finish that breakfast, and I want to tell you about a key element of this training program: self-coaching.

Yes, self-coaching. Pretty soon, two more days from now, you'll be back home, on your own. Given the structure and individualization of this program, you'll have a good sense about what you should do. It's important to try to stick to it as best as you can. But no coach, nor any book, can foresee every situation and answer every question you'll have. And that's okay. That's good. Even my personal clients, whom I speak to on a daily/weekly basis, have to adjust their program for themselves, measuring what works with their schedules and their bodies.

Embrace self-coaching. Life gets in the way. Sometimes you're sick. Sometimes work can take you out of your routine. Sometimes family commitments interfere. Sometimes you just don't bring it to the trail that day. Sometimes you feel like you can push harder. Sometimes you feel like you can't. That's all okay. That's human. It's not a perfect world, and even if it were, everybody realizes his or her best in different ways. So you have to take some ownership of your training and self-coach. Already, you've begun to be aware over the past few days of how that works. For instance, in strength training, I told you to manipulate the number of sets/reps based on your ability—and time availability. Same with your foundation program, where you decide for yourself at the beginning of the schedule whether you're able to train six days a week, or how many interval reps to perform. Same with nutrition and deciding on your mission statement.

By its very nature, self-coaching requires you to make adjustments on your own. So there's no set of rules on how to do it. That said, here are some broad parameters and pointed tips that might help you along the way:

1. Workouts (sequence): Remember that all the workouts and exercises have a purpose, whether easy or difficult. Follow the sequence of your weekly schedule, and keep to the assigned workouts and intensity. This sequence and spacing of runs is very important, as they take into account the training effect and your recovery needs on a daily, weekly, and monthly basis. Everything has a purpose. Everything works together. As a general rule, if you have to miss one to two runs during the week, that's okay; carry on with the program that week, and don't try to make up the missed workouts. If you miss more than two workouts in a week, it's best to repeat the week, moving the whole schedule forward. Do not shuffle workouts around and mess with the sequence.

2. Listen and be smart: No one knows your body better than you do. Sometimes you will need to back off on a run or take the day off, either because you simply don't feel great, or maybe you felt a slight pull in the hamstring during your last run. Listen to your body and understand your situation. Whether because of illness or just not feeling "right," I instruct my athletes to take the day off—or at the least, make the day an easy one. But also understand, there's a difference between feeling "off" or sick versus just not wanting to do a run and workout. Be aware of this difference. Also be patient. Many times, it's easy to be amped up at the beginning of the program and want to do more than scheduled. Pull in the reins and pace yourself throughout each week, each month. Just like in a race, you do not want to start out too fast and burn out at the end. Trust the process.

3. Consistency: When it comes to improvement and proper fitness, consistency is huge. Use this as motivation to get runs in when you can, even if you don't feel like getting out the door. One, you will feel better once you do, and these days go a long way toward offsetting those that come when life, injury, or illness gets in the way. Because it will, so always do what you have time to do, even if it is much less than what is scheduled. Running easily for thirty minutes is better than not doing anything because you can't fit in the sixty-minute scheduled run. Let me repeat: Something is better than nothing. Many times athletes will think that if they do not have time for the entire workout, the day's a wash and it's not worth doing even part of it. Not true! Twenty to thirty minutes goes a long way toward being consistent.

4. Log workouts: Write down what you do every day. Again and again I've seen in my coaching, whether of beginning runners or elites, that those who religiously log their workouts achieve more success. There's just something about that personal accountability, and the reward you get from logging what you did each day, that leads to great performances. Because of this, I require all my athletes to log their workouts. If you enjoy the techie way, there're many online run log systems out there. Or do it old-school: Keep a journal; jot down what you did that day, and add a few comments about the run, how long, where, how you felt, what you learned, and what you were aware of along the way.

5. Difficulty: During the program, things will get tough and challenging. Don't confuse this difficulty with some failure of yours. Our muscles and body need to be pushed to improve. Trust me; I understand the feeling, the frustration you might experience, the "It's so hard. . . . It shouldn't be this hard. . . . I can't do this. . . ." When you are having these feelings, these thoughts, stop and recognize them. Then start to see difficulty as an opportunity to get better, physically and mentally.

6. Nutrition: Again and again I tell my athletes, "You are only one good choice away from righting the ship." If you have found that you have made a few bad choices that do not reflect your mission statement, simply focus on making a good choice the next meal.

YOUR RUNNING PERSONALITY

As a coach, I've found it crucial to understand the personality—the running personality, if you will—of the athletes I'm working with. Just as I study and make notes to myself about such physical things as a runner's stride and arm carriage, flexibility and muscle balance, so too do I make note of psychological aspects of the athlete that I observe. These elements aren't set in stone, and they certainly don't predetermine everything, but they can help me figure out the best approach to working with that runner.

What kind of runner are you? See if any of the four types below fits you best; then give some thought to my tips on the best self-coaching approach given your personality.

1. The Perfectionist

- *Traits*—Detail-oriented. Plans all workouts and races to the mile and the minute. Loves schedules and lists. A meticulous record keeper. Often dependent upon a coach.
- *Motivation*—Measurable improvement and mastery. Perfectionists really want to know that they are improving, and gain as much knowledge as possible and do everything they can to improve, hitting all the checkpoints. They get excited about new challenges by researching and learning as much as possible.
- *Stress*—Weather, illness, injury; any interruption to training, any change to plans. Needs to listen to the body during stressful times and be okay with taking a day off when one is not scheduled. Perfectionists can sometimes get frustrated with challenges that they are not used to, which can give them a feeling of failure. They can get hung up on needing to know how things will work out and what the outcomes will be for their training or racing.
- *Self-coaching approach*—This kind of runner needs to learn that listening to the body is as important as following the schedule. Perfectionists have to learn to let go occasionally and introduce variations into the plan and rejuvenation time to avoid plateaus. They need to embrace the unexpected and new challenges for the body and mind.

2. The Charger

- *Traits*—Take-charge approach. Loves the challenge of races or workouts. Will jump into either with or without conventional preparation.
- *Motivation*—Results; making the next leap. Enjoys the social aspects of the next challenge, thinking big and being in the middle of it all.
- *Stress*—Delays; recovery time; too much step-by-step; "If you're not getting better, you're getting worse!"
- *Self-coaching approach*—This kind of runner needs frequent challenges, but these should be layered in base and foundational work so that chargers' abilities keep improving. They need to guard against overwork. They need to embrace the benefits of following some structure so they do not do too much too soon.

3. The Social Strider

- *Traits*—Thrives on interaction with training partners and a group. Performance varies in keeping with companions'.
- *Motivation*—Relationships and camaraderie. Sense of belonging.
- *Stress*—A competitive atmosphere. A focus on performance.
- *Self-coaching approach*—This type of runner needs to define the personal goals that go beyond group interaction. Social striders can do well paired with a training partner who can push their performance level. They need a workout that blends in enough solo running. Encourage training partners to conduct a group workout. Communicate training needs to partners and be creative in fitting in personal workouts within a group setting.

4. The Free Spirit

- *Traits*—The adventurer. Creative and likes diversity and new challenges. Appreciates running for more than just the competitive and fitness aspects. Might possess a combination of traits of the other types.
- *Motivation*—The immediate physical and emotional sensations of running. New experiences. Commitment. The entire process of creating new adventures, and the training and prep that go into it. Enjoys the process as much as the outcome or success. Free spirits are motivated by diversity.
- *Stress*—Routine. Stressful or hectic life demands that take them away from being able to run consistently.
- *Self-coaching approach*—This runner needs to build in diversions through the use of varied routes, multiple training partners, training "play and adventure." Free spirits can use special events, challenges, and races to serve as motivation to adhering to some kind of training structure and focus.

Fun, right—and maybe a little scary—to think of yourself as one of these types? But this kind of recognition and self-awareness will help you along the way. So, now you have a good idea of how to work everything together—and how to guide yourself. Let me pay the check, and we'll get out there on the trail, where we'll have time to go deeper into awareness (essential to self-coaching) and begin the journey to discovering your Cool Impossible.

8

ATHLETICISM = AWARENESS

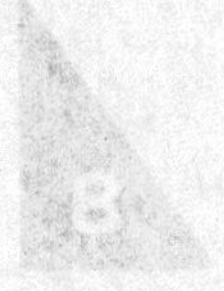

ON LEAVING THE Bunnery, we take my truck and head west from Jackson, across the Snake River and toward Teton Pass. It's a steep, winding road, and you'll see some road cyclists zipping down it like flashes of light.

During the winter, the surrounding mountainsides are a backcountry skiing paradise. As the sun rises, many in Jackson will head out for "dawn patrol." They leave their cars at the top of Teton Pass. Boots on, skis lashed to their backs, they hike up seventeen hundred vertical feet, then ski the fresh powder down through the trees, hitchhike back up to the car with their gear, and finally head off to work. Not bad for a morning, right?

Today's a bit of a drive, but I promise it's worth the jaunt. We have a long trail run up to a ridge beside Taylor Mountain, up to ten thousand feet for your legs and lungs to enjoy. There will be more than enough time for me to stride at your side, speaking of why and how we must train our minds to realize our Cool Impossible. Try not to let your thoughts wander—not yet, anyway. There's some heavy stuff in here, real brain-twisting stuff, so I ask you to pay close attention, and keep faith that I'm leading you on the right path, both literally and figuratively.

Let's hit it. We start off at the Coal Creek Trailhead. Along the way, watch for bears, and make sure you keep your eyes on the path. A lot of tree roots and stones to avoid. Stay aware, keenly aware.

As an athlete and coach, I've always believed in training the mind as much as the body. I've known, even intuitively as a kid, of the importance of the mind-body connection in sports performance—and life performance. By focusing on this connection, I've achieved many of my own ambitions—as have my athletes. So can you.

Experience and time can be excellent teachers for a coach. Over thousands of hours training various people, I've learned to see the good and bad in how my athletes move. It's become instinctive for me now. The same goes for how my athletes think. I train good and bad thinkers: those who see no walls and those who see them at every turn. Every day I see how this impacts their training sessions and, ultimately, of course, their overall race performances.

The mental leads the physical; it's clear. Over and over again, I've seen a lesser physical athlete with a fierce mental attitude—someone who is aware of his thinking and clear in his ambitions, and doesn't interpret difficulty as failure—wipe from the track an athlete who is more physically talented but also crippled by fear, doubts, and uncertainty about his goals. Our bodies react to emotions and what we tell ourselves, and yet more often than not, we're not even conscious of what we're telling our bodies, much less careful and directed about it.

Through time, I've become able to pick apart an athlete's mental weakness as easily as his or her run form mechanics. This isn't rocket science, nor clairvoyance; it's simply awareness. If you listen closely to how a runner talks—whether of tough runs, his latest race, during training, or competition—his interior world is revealed. This talk, his or her thoughts, have turned into habits, in the same way one acquires bad running form. Over time, these "thought habits," good and bad, build on themselves and, in the eyes of the athlete, become truths. Listen to how other runners talk, just as I asked you to watch how others run. You can learn to see the problems and strengths in their running form, and you can start to hear how their thoughts help and hurt their performance. There's much to learn.

The truth is, most of us have lost that sense of boundless possibility we once knew so easily as children. We simply know too much—or so we think—and therefore we stop ourselves before we even make the attempt at our ambitions.

No more, I say.

As Aldous Huxley said, "Experience is not what happens to you; it's what you do with what happens to you." There's great insight there, and I'd like to put my own spin on it. I say, "It is not important what we think; it's important what we do with what we think."

What's beautiful is that we can learn how to train our minds the same as we can our legs, lungs, and heart. I've developed a system that will allow you to not only manage your fears, but benefit from them. There are methods, through visualizations, mantras, and rituals, that will empower you to identify and realize your Cool Impossible. Many of my athletes have discovered newfound power in these lessons and have taken them to do everything from qualifying for the Boston Marathon to winning world championships. That personal best, that ultramarathon, that big race, whether on the track or in life—they are all within reach for you as well.

First, though, must come more understanding.

THE PERILS AND POWER OF OUR THOUGHTS

You're striding well. Nice forefoot strike, and you've handled those early switchbacks like a champ. Feel how you used that strength in your feet, how your body stabilized. Now we have a long, even stretch clear through the pines. But there's a chill. Fall's coming soon. Those shrub oaks will turn a nice red, the aspens yellow. Soon enough it'll be ski season, these trails buried in snow too deep to run; that's for sure.

If you like to hit the slopes, though, you'll see how much the physical athleticism you've developed pays off in other sports as well.

Let's stick to this one for now, and I have a statement to make: If you so choose, you can become the runner you fantasize about being. I'm talking any fantasy, even 150-mile ultramarathons. Whoa, don't pitch off the side of the trail. Stay steady. I haven't lost it. Now, I make that remark to prove a point. Besides questioning my sanity, I bet you asked yourself a question (right after, "Is Eric suffering altitude sickness?"), because most of us go quickly to the same question when a goal is set before us.

Can I do it?

If I tried to run a 150-mile race, where would my legs crumble; when would I go delirious; at what mile would my heart explode? I joke a little, but the point is important. We, as human beings, want to know the outcome of things before we even set on the trail to do them. We have an innate desire to know the answer to "What if?" Yet at the start of any adventure, it's impossible to know what will happen. None of us owns a crystal ball, and if we did, I'm pretty sure it wouldn't help anyway. There are no guarantees for any outcome. So why not start simply for the adventure of it all?

Unless you've run an ultramarathon already—or come close—I suspect that your response to my statement that you could run a 150-miler was simply "No, I can't." You saw the outcome. You predicted you'd collapse around mile ten, twenty, thirty, forty—wherever. Of course, depending on your level of fitness and running experience, you might well have the same response if I said you can run a 10K or half marathon.

This kind of thinking, this need to know, often dictates what we take on and try to accomplish. Since we can't know the future, we more often than not decide this or that ambition is beyond our reach. In a way, it's a safety mechanism to prevent ourselves from failing. To avoid it, we either aim too low in our goals or never venture down the road to achieving the big ones—or both.

Why? Because we fear both failure and the unknown. Fear is a powerful motivating force. And it comes in many shapes and sizes, from internal demons to external threats. Most of our fears emerge from experience. You say, "I want to run a marathon, but in the past, I've found that after mile five of any run, my hip begins to hurt." If that's the kind of response you have, I suspect you see only failure in an attempt to run a marathon. Because you're not sure you can do it, and you're afraid you'll have pain if you try, you assume you can't. But that assumption is just an expression of your need to know the outcome. Since you can't know the future, you're trying to predict it through your previous experiences. The need to know manipulates your thinking into stopping you from even trying the marathon. Over time, you don't even venture the "need-to-know" question any longer. You simply begin to believe that the goal is impossible. Fear transforms into belief. It's a self-perpetuating cycle that begins and ends in our minds.

I see you smiling. What all this means, wonderfully, is that our thinking, our fear of failure and the unknown, is not real. It's merely a fabrication of our minds, a side effect of past experiences or "made-up" fear. We often see our thinking as undeniable truth. But it's not. We make our thoughts. And they are only as real as we allow them to be. Begin looking at your thoughts as just another part of your body, like your leg or arm. You have awareness now about your forefoot strike, and I want you to have the same mindfulness of how your thoughts are separate from you and who you are.

Here's the real power in this understanding: If our thoughts are not reality and are only what we make them, then we can create good stories as well as bad stories. We have a choice. We can set whatever ending we want in our minds: crossing the finish line, running a personal best. Our thinking, when stuck in a bad story, becomes an obstacle. Our thinking, when playing a good story, becomes a tool of incredible use. If bad thoughts are based on bad past experiences, then we can also look to the past and find good experiences to shape good thoughts to help us with future outcomes.

Before you doubt your ability to banish all negative thoughts, stop. That is not what I'm asking you to do. There is no pill, no method of training your mind, to fill yourself with only happy, good stories that lead you to success. There will always be fears, because we will always have a ton of unknowns. The point is not to expect them to vanish. We want to embrace our fears, realize they are not real, and then move past them to act on our Cool Impossible.

Many people believe that elite athletes are free of negative thoughts. Somehow they are superhuman, outside the bounds of us mere mortals. I've known many such "superhumans," and they have fears and doubts equal to your own. They only deal with them differently, often in ways that turn them into an advantage.

Instead of trying to banish your fears and the bad stories they tell, do something different. Be aware of them, identify them for what they are—only thoughts—and no matter what, keep moving forward. If you can do this, while creating good stories of your own, then you've given yourself the ability to achieve and live the life you want to live.

IN THE FLOW

Rah! Rah! Inspirational stuff! I hope you find it so—even if you aren't convinced. I don't expect you to be. Yet. The proof is in the pudding. You need to see it work for yourself. Otherwise, these are only words. You'll forget them without practice and execution, same as my lessons on your running form. It's one thing to tell you how to run, another for you to work at it day after day, solidifying your form, watching yourself gain speed and endurance. You should deal the same way with your thoughts. Can you begin to conceptualize now that if we separate our actions from our thoughts, then anything is possible?

Slow it down a little. I'm not sure whether you noticed, but you really revved up your pace down the trail during all that talk of overcoming fears, creating your own good stories. There's a great deal of empowerment there, particularly as you begin to see how your body "listens" to your thoughts.

I first experienced this connection as a boy. The night before a Little

League game, I was all fired up. There were two things I knew: One, I feared whiffing at bat and striking out. Two, I wanted desperately to hit a home run. Instead of focusing on the first, I thought most of the second. I thought about how I'd step into the box, the pitch would come, and *bam*—with the crack of ball against bat, I'd nail one over the left fielder, out past the wall. Gone, baby, gone. Before bed, I told my mother that was exactly what would happen the next day. Guess what? It did; that ball sailed from my bat like it never had before.

How did this happen? What is this connection between mind and body? How did I move past my fears and find myself in a place where this was possible? Was it just dumb luck, a too-slow pitch, and a brisk wind?

At thirteen years old, I didn't have any of these answers, but what I did recognize as true even at that age was that my thoughts had helped create and determine my future performance outcome.

Okay, I'm getting ahead of myself. With my athletes, and in my own life, I've seen how impactful our minds can be in realizing our goals, and I want to get you on that path as quickly as possible.

Let's take it even slower. You'll wear yourself out trying to over-stride these hills. Let the trail come to you, and keep stepping over those imaginary logs. I want to give you a little more Eric Orton philosophy, but it's soon layered with practical steps, things you can start to do, even now as we run.

I hope you understand how our thoughts, fabricated though they are, are connected to our actions. They turn around and around together, feeding each other in a cycle, both positively and negatively, depending on the stories we are telling. You can break this cycle, control it, and the key is awareness.

On the first day we worked on the fundamentals of form, there was a moment, I could tell, when you were what I like to call completely "in the flow." You were running around the track at a slow pace, focused on your forefoot strike, smooth breathing, knee drive, bow-and-arrow push-off on the straight leg, and the movement of your arms. From the look on your face, nothing else was entering your mind. You were in the present; all fears of whether you had the strength or ability were gone. At that moment, I'm sure time seemed to slow down for you. Distance, weariness meant nothing. Awareness had brought you in the flow, and it was beautiful.

Instead of focusing on what our body is doing, we can turn this same level of awareness onto what is going on in our head, and it will free us from fear and empower us to choose the future we want.

How? Why? What?

Whether you know it or not, your mind is constantly churning through thoughts, interpreting the world around you, often based on past experience. In a way, without even being aware, you're constantly talking to yourself. Often this talk is negative: you trying to gauge an outcome and your inability then to reach it. As I've said, this then leads you to quit or lower your ambitions. This is happening all the time, most often subconsciously, because the thought patterns are so ingrained.

Now, as soon as you're aware of these thoughts, as soon as you tune in to this chatter, it stops. Now you're in the flow, no longer predicting some future or defining the same by the past. Instead of fabricating more thoughts, you can now evaluate them for what they are: only stories that you made up. They're not real. Once you have this awareness, then you can make a choice about what you want to do—a choice based not on fear but rather on your goals. You're no longer reacting to your thoughts; you're acting on your wishes free of them.

Let me give you an example of how this played out with one of my athletes on a small level. Then, through some exercises with you, I'll show you how it works personally for you.

Remember the scorpion exercise in the strength program? A few years back, I had a runner from Pennsylvania come out to visit me for some training. He was reasonably athletic, reasonably fit, about average for the marathoners you see at the starting line. Well, he was having knee pain and wanted to ramp up his abilities, maybe even do an ultra. It was clear he had some instability, range of motion, and gluteus medius issues, but nothing insurmountable.

We worked through the first stages of the slant board exercises. All was fine. Then we hit the dynamic movements with the Fitball. On scorpion, the first time he tried to rotate his hips and bend the knee back to his opposite arm, boom, he was on the floor. He tried again, didn't fall, but the form was all over the place. He was competitive, tried again and again, but he never got it right. I could see his frustration, and he made it clear later. We moved on.

Two days later, we were working through the program again, and we came to the scorpion. He wanted to skip it, try later, maybe months later, when he felt like he had developed some more athleticism. Okay, I said, but first, I told him to sit down. He gave me a strange look. I gave him a blank one back. He closed his eyes. Then I asked him to focus on the chatter going on in his head about the scorpion.

"Don't judge the thoughts," I told him. "They're just thoughts. Negative ones don't make you bad. We all have them. Just be aware of them."

He spilled: "I'm thinking, 'I don't need this exercise. My quads are too tight. This won't make me a better runner. I'll put in the motions, but this will never happen.'"

Then I asked him to think about why he was having these thoughts. Where did they come from? He was honest. He said he was supercompetitive, and he'd rather not look like a fool, unable to do what others obviously could.

And there, *boom*, he was aware of his thoughts. He had stopped spinning them in his mind, allowing them to defeat him. His frustration was caused by his fear of failing. Can you see that in yourself?

I told him, "Who cares if you can't do scorpion now? Will you try? Will you work toward doing it? You can keep to your bad thoughts or make new ones that say, 'I don't stink at this; it's meant to be hard.' Maybe start with doing just one right, and how great it would be in a few months to do ten."

He had a choice now, one based on awareness, rather than a reaction to his fears of looking silly in front of me. It helped him get started. A lot of time has passed, and he's a scorpion master now, this athlete. It was a small thing for him, really. There are other exercises that would have had the same benefit as scorpion. I could have given him those to do. But the point was for him to listen to the thoughts going on in his head, to know they were just thoughts and not real, to understand how they were affecting actions, and to find a way to be in the flow, in the present, making informed choices.

Remember the Great Gazoo from *The Flintstones*? He was that little floating green-skinned alien with the big helmet who was constantly whispering in Fred's ear, telling him one thing or another. It may sound ridiculous, but in a way, we all have our own Gazoo who's providing this internal dialogue day to day, throughout our life, that nobody else can see. If we allow our Gazoo to make our decisions for us, then we're living unaware, and more times than not allowing our fears to direct our lives. Be aware of your Gazoo, stop his voice, and choose a path forward based on your big-picture goals rather than on your fears.

Begin this by listening to your own thoughts; see how much your actions are based on them. Test this philosophy now, and over the next few days.

Really, what's going on right this second on the Coal Creek trail? We've come down into a mountain meadow; butterflies swirl around us by the score. We're more than halfway to the ridge. Yes, that ridge, the one that looks almost straight up—that's where we're heading.

You're breathing heavily, even at this slower pace. Are you thinking you're tired, and you don't know how you'll continue running for another fifteen hundred feet of vertical? Yup, that's what you are doing today, four miles up and thirty-three hundred feet of climbing. Are you worried about not being able to keep up with me, needing to take more breaks? Do you think you might just not make it at all?

Examine these thoughts, because they are fears about outcomes. You can't know for sure whether you'll need to walk the last stretch to the ridge. But this worry is based on your need to know. Break the cycle of those thoughts by being aware of the now. Check your pace, your breathing, form, foot strike; self-evaluate. Focus on what you can do now versus what will happen as we begin those switchbacks up to the ridge. The choice you have now, this moment, is how you will run the next fifty feet. Savor the quest, not the finish.

Be Chris Sharma. Heard the name? He's one of the world's best climbers. On one route in Spain, he made one hundred unsuccessful tries before reaching the top. One hundred attempts, one route, no ropes, and every time he failed he would fall thirty to forty feet into deep water below. Chris fell in love with seeing how far along the route he could get each time. He fell in love with what climbers call the "project," the present effort. Think of Chris Sharma whenever the fear of finishing a race or training session comes into your mind. Think of Chris, and refocus on your foot hitting the ground for your next step.

Flashing forward, when you work on your twenty-day detox, pay attention to your thoughts as well. Again, don't judge them, right or wrong; just pay attention to what you're telling yourself. Write them down on a piece of paper if that helps. Start to see how emotions, beliefs, feelings come out through our thinking when we try to make good food choices. This is particularly heightened during the detox, because it's focused, structured, and, well, frankly, tough.

Are you saying, "This isn't worth it," or, "I've always done fine on my diet," or, "This is crazy; I can't maintain this for three weeks; life's too busy; I can't be so picky at restaurants. Don't I deserve a sweet? What would it hurt?"

Can you "see" these thoughts, be aware of them as just that, thoughts, not as truths? Do you notice how they stop and lose their power once you're aware and identifying them? Then you can make a choice. Being your best is just a choice.

Start to play a game with yourself: See how quickly you catch these thoughts throughout the day. Don't worry; you're not crazy with all these voices whirling around in your head. Everyone has that inner dialogue. But not everyone is aware enough to break the cycle of its power. The important thing is not to want to do away with your bad thoughts—or even change them. You will have them—the best of us do—but you can learn to look for them, listen to yourself, realize they're just thoughts, and that they have no impact on your actions and who you really are—unless you allow it.

Dive deeper now. Have your own conversation with them. "I wonder why I'm thinking that? Why do I think I need pizza? Why don't I want to go for a run today? Why do I feel like I have to run today when it's my day off?" Observe your thoughts and keep moving right through them. Don't allow them to alter your actions, or what you know you need to do to reach your goals for the day and the days beyond.

The more you do this, the more you'll be in the flow. As I said, make it a game, this listening to your thoughts, your fears. "Oh, there it is again," say to yourself. It's okay if the bad stories keep returning; they will. What's important is that you recognize them for what they are. You'll get better at this. It's no different from working a muscle, this awareness of your thoughts and moving past them. You'll get stronger.

You look pretty strong now, taking that last fifty feet of calf-burning, lung-searing incline to the ridge. You're in the flow.

Now, how many times have you heard—and hopefully felt—that you were "in the zone" or experiencing a "runner's high"? You know: that feeling, in a race or intense run, that there was nothing you could do wrong. Everything fell into place. You could see everything, everyone, what you had done, and what you needed to do. You were unstoppable, yet you made no judgment about that; nor did you revel in it. You were simply at peace, at one with what you were doing, and you could not miss. The basketball net was somehow wider. Your competitors were slower. You anticipated their moves and knew where the ball was going long before it got there. You were strong, fast, focused, and full of energy, with effortless breathing, your muscles fresh as when you started. The world, everything outside the field or track or stadium, was gone. You were in the moment, yet above it as well.

Beautiful, right? Sublime. We all love being in the zone. Yet it is a mystery how to reach this perfect place. So much goes into it, and its discovery is unpredictable and often frustratingly elusive. You're peaking athletically. You capture some early success that spikes your confidence. You find yourself charged by the crowd or a word of support from a friend. These things, many others, may contribute to your realizing that special window of ability.

But I would argue that one element is always there, always necessary: being in the flow. Many people sloppily use these terms interchangeably, but for me being in the zone is not the same as being in the flow. In fact, it's being in the flow that enables and is a prerequisite to achieving the zone. Being in the flow means being fully attentive to the present moment, to your foot hitting the ground for your next stride, your breathing, your stance, your body in motion—nothing else. The past, the future, they are nothing. As soon as we are aware of what we are doing or thinking, our external thoughts stop. Time slows because of this heightened awareness. You feel effortless and relaxed. Once you're there, truly there, you can find yourself in the zone, when all your abilities, mental and physical, come together so perfectly that you seem to be able to do everything and anything.

The beauty of being in the flow is that, with practice, it is a state you can reach every hour of every day. You can be focused on the now in every run, every workout.

CREATE YOUR COOL IMPOSSIBLE

Sit down on that boulder. Take a while to soak in that view, just like that hawk circling down below. Yes, below. You're above where hawks fly, ten thousand feet high. Mountains in every direction. Long rows of pines. Breathe that air, clear as that blue sky. You did a great run up here. Good work staying in the flow.

From the look in your eyes, you're having a bit of a freebie. Breathe; take a drink of water. "Freebie?" That's what we out here in Jackson Hole like to call light-headedness from the altitude—cheaper than bellying up to the bar.

While I've got you taking in the beauty, I want to talk about how awareness can lead us to knowing what we want. What I'm about to tell you is a bit heavy, so take it in slowly; chew on it well. Here goes: If our past experiences influence our thinking in the present, and this thinking influences the actions we will take in the future, then . . . and here it is . . . our thinking in the present creates the future.

That's the philosophy, but now let's focus on how to perceive and realize the future you want. Creating your Cool Impossible will be fun, and we're in the perfect spot for you to let your mind wander. This is the first step to creating what we want. I like to call it daydreaming, but with a caveat: You have to rid yourself of any negative perceptions of that word. We are not talking about staring out the window, mind empty, eyes blank. What I'm talking about is daydreaming of a different type. It's a journey into your mind, but one where you take whatever paths come along the way. Don't be rigid with a map, a certain destination, not yet.

You can start to daydream here on the ridge, but I want you to do it anytime you have a moment of freedom from daily life. I like to daydream on long runs, while listening to music or sitting at home drinking my morning coffee or evening tea. Simply be in a place where interruptions are at a minimum. Close your eyes or keep them open; be in a public place or a private one; cross your legs or not—do what makes you comfortable.

Now, let your mind let go of everything present and begin thinking of a goal you want to accomplish with your running. Anything you want. Start fantasizing. Maybe it's to run the Grand Canyon, or your first 10K or hundred-miler; maybe it's to qualify for the Boston Marathon or the Olympic Trials, or to race some wicked fast time.

Get so relaxed, so at ease that questions of whether this is possible for you to accomplish are of no consequence. They will not stop your dreaming. Of course, thoughts will creep in, negative ones, no doubt, but acknowledge them and keep dreaming. Go big here. Go for the biggest, craziest, coolest dream you could imagine for yourself. I want you so excited about this dream that goose bumps run up your arm. Literally. The more excited you get, the better. Just smile as you create this Cool Impossible, because we don't care whether it will happen. Just create the ultimate fantasy for yourself.

Continue letting your mind wander; allow your thoughts to jump around and take you in different directions. Have fun. No judgments. Try as best you can to shoot for a measurable goal instead of an emotion or state of being. You might dream, "I want to feel healthy." That's great, but go further. What specific goal will make you feel you've reached a level of healthfulness that you never imagined for yourself before? Keep going—what makes you so excited; what ambition rocks your world?

In the next days—or weeks and months, as long as it takes—keep daydreaming. Learn to love and have fun with the experience. No rules. Daydream your coolest life or race or whatever. Allow your mind to drift where it takes you. Don't push yourself toward the "right" thing. Trust your instincts. When your Cool Impossible—for that's what you'll find through this experience—comes to you, you will know it. If it's a long-term goal, great. If it's more immediate, great. Does one build on the other? Wonderful. You can have several Cool Impossibles going at once. Like I said, no rules. Learn to love this, because now all this creation can be so fun, it's a game at life, a game for life—how big can you make life for yourself?

Years ago, I came to my own Cool Impossible while allowing my mind to wander. And my dream is to have one runner in every household in America, and beyond. I want to spread the joy and health benefits that come with running to everyone in the world. It's a big goal; some would say impossible. Perfect. It's my dream, and I'm living it.

Once you've found yours, start to feel how excited you become when thinking about it. Awesome, right? And if you feel some fear, that's worth getting excited about as well. Do you know why?

Because fear is a measure of things. It means your Cool Impossible is significant to you. It means you've created the biggest, baddest goal possible for yourself. It means it has value. I always like to say—so maybe you've heard it already—"If it seems impossible, it might be worth doing." Fear is a good signal, and as long as we keep it from leading our actions, then it can be a positive force in our lives. If you're a little anxious, nervous, fearful about your ambitions—or even in the moment—then you're likely creating the life, the Cool Impossible you want. If you think about it, fear is necessary for great things, impossible things. I'm not interested in "no fear" or fearlessness. No, thanks. I say more fear—bring it on. Embrace it. Love it.

Is any Cool Impossible attainable, then? It's the obvious next question, and one I'm asked again and again. If you're honest with yourself and follow your daydreams intuitively, then I believe the answer is yes. For instance, I don't sit awake at night, allowing my mind to wander, and find myself imagining sitting in the Oval Office, ruler of the free world. Nor do I see myself winning Olympic gold in the shot put. These two ambitions, and many others that people might find perfectly reasonable for themselves, never enter my consciousness. But one runner in every household? Yes, for me that's an idea worth thinking about.

Once you have created your true Cool Impossible, you're ready to begin practicing the tactics to realize it.

TRAINING YOUR MIND

Start back down the ridge with me. Down these inclines, stutter your steps sideways. On this steep slope, there's lots of loose dirt and rocks that are a sure recipe for a fall. Once we get a bit of the way down, we'll run again. Remember, imagine you're riding a bike as you go downhill. It took us an hour to get up, but it will be half that coming down. Less effort, so you'll have time to take in more of the scenery. When those aspens turn bright yellow in the fall, they make the hillsides look like they're painted gold. That east-facing cliff to your right is an epic ski line in winter.

I believe being an athlete is a choice, and that we all can be athletes, regardless of natural ability. It is a mind-set, a lifestyle, a decision. As we make our descent, I want you to imagine yourself doing the techniques I'm about to tell you about to train your athletic mind. Together mantras, rituals, and visualizations are fundamental to athletic performance and realizing your goals on a day-to-day basis, as fundamental as form or strength. I only ask that you try it for yourself; work at this level of awareness for several months.

See the difference in your performance and how it can reshape your mind-set.

The first step of the three is to develop a mantra.

1. Mantras

In sports performance tradition, a mantra is a word or collection of words that are repeated frequently and help focus an individual's concentration and performance. Most if not all high-performing athletes use them consciously or subconsciously. I personally recommend you use a mantra to call yourself back into the flow. Your mantra is a tool to focus your mind and disarm any negative thoughts that will try to sabotage you.

I recommend you pick a mantra that is three words that describe qualities you must have to accomplish your goal. Instead of simply drawing these from a hat, it's best to identify the three by asking yourself what obstacles stand in the way of your achieving your Cool Impossible. Look deep inside yourself and examine your fears and the negative thoughts that you anticipate will arise once you're moving down the road to your goal.

Some examples:

- My schedule is too busy. I don't have time to train.
- I just don't have the innate talent.
- I am too old, too young, too out of shape.
- People think I'm crazy to be working out this much.
- This is a silly midlife crisis. I should get a red convertible instead.
- My injuries will rear their ugly heads again.
- Money will get in the way.
- My strongest, fastest days are behind me.

Make this list as long and detailed as you can. Really delve deep into your mind; expose your dark fears to the light of day. Write them down. Once you finish this list, ask yourself what three qualities or feelings you need to overcome and dispel these fears whenever they arise (for it won't be just once). Typically these words tend to be emotional states, or often better yet, action words that will empower you in those tough moments—the last leg of a race, the middle of a long training session, the early cold morning when you want to stay in bed. Your mantra is meant to focus you when you're having trouble staying in the flow, when your doubts and fears are running rampant.

Further, your three mantra words should evoke a reaction, a physical and emotional one. They should resonate within you almost viscerally. You might find they come from characteristics you respect in other athletes, or they're traits to succeed that you always felt you lacked—but always wanted. Last, but most obviously, they should be positive.

As examples, here're several mantra words I've known my athletes to use:

- Persistent
- Confident
- Indomitable
- Independent
- Strong
- Efficient
- Resourceful
- Just go
- Patient
- Spirit
- Willful

Drawing from these, your three-word mantra might be: "Strong, independent, persistent." Or you can turn the mantra into a statement, but if you do that, remember it should still be based on the three words. For instance, your mantra could be, "I am strong, independent, and always persistent." Spend time creating your mantra, testing out what feelings you really want and need.

Once you find your mantra, write it down in big block letters. You're ready to pair it with the second step to training your mind: a ritual.

2. Ritual

No doubt you've used rituals in your own life already, whether in preparing to take a test, interview for a job, or go into a race. You've seen them too, probably lots of times without even knowing it. How many athletes have you seen who wear the same shorts or socks before a race? That's a ritual. Or the pitcher who jumps over the foul-ball line every time before heading to the mound. Ritual. In my football days, once I was mentally ready for a game, I put on my helmet and never took it off until the final whistle. Ritual. When waiting for a punt or kickoff return, I hopped on each foot five times before the kick. Ritual.

Like mantras, rituals act to center us, to trigger focus in our minds, to bring us into the flow. When paired with the mantra, they are even more effective. To create your ritual, think of something that is easy to do, subtle, and can be performed anytime, anywhere, without being distracting to yourself or others or requiring undue effort. You might need to do this ritual while running or in a busy place, whenever the need arises for you to get in the flow to perform and return your awareness to your goals at hand.

I blink my eyes three times. That's my ritual. I like to pair the three words of my mantra with three acts in my ritual. You could tap your hand three times against your leg. Snap your fingers. Curl your toes. Clench and unclench your fist. Rub your ear three times. You get the idea. Once you have a mantra and a ritual, now we add visualization to this powerful brew.

3. Visualization

As you now know, I'm a big believer in creating something in your mind's eye. It is remarkable to me that people don't do it more. They're missing out on so much unused power.

Okay, so there are many ways to use visualization. I'll begin with its ability to connect emotion to our mantra and ritual, magnifying their effect. This works because emotion is a powerful motivator for both our bodies and minds. Throughout I'll refer to this visualization technique as finding your flow state, because that's what it'll help you do.

Visualization—Warming Up to Navigate Your Mind's Pathways

The more you practice visualization, the better at it you get. In addition to doing your visualization to empower your mantra and ritual, I recommend practicing visualization just to empower your mind. Think of it as strength and endurance training for your brain.

It's best to do your visualizations at home in a quiet room free of distractions. Early morning, when I'm at my most alert, is my favorite time, but find your own. This is a warm-up, a way to practice visualizing your mind's pathways. Close your eyes, breathe normally, and take yourself back to a moment in the previous week, one of some significance or eventfulness. It could be a long run, a romantic dinner, a celebration at work. Bring yourself right back to that day as an observer. Note the surroundings, the mood. Are you smiling, laughing? Is it loud or quiet? Relive that moment. Now move to another day, perhaps yesterday. Put yourself right back there in a specific moment in that day. See it, feel it, hear it. Keep traveling on your mind's pathway, but now project forward; visualize two days from now. Imagine what you will do, how you'll dress, whom you'll see. Maybe focus on that long run you have planned with friends, or a race. Make it come alive. Finally, move back to today, this moment; open your eyes.

Now, your flow state is a moment in your past when you feel you had the qualities of your mantra. Say, when you were at your strongest, most independent and persistent. Think back to a time or an event when you displayed those traits. Don't worry about how far back you need to go, as long as that moment is vivid and detailed in your memory. Take yourself back there, close your eyes, and follow the pathways of your mind to that time. Once there, relive it; make it as real as you can by remembering as many details as you can. Hear the noises. See the people, the scene. Experience this moment as it happened. And most of all, sense how good you felt about yourself; savor how strong, independent, persistent you were at that moment. Take as long as you need to get there; enjoy that time again. While you're there, notice how your memories are creating emotions by revisiting this experience. Notice how the visualization of something in the past is giving you real, immediate feelings in the present.

When this past moment is vivid in your mind's eye, when you can feel the same emotions you experienced at that time in your body now again, say your mantra and do your ritual, all together. Do this several times, if you want. When you feel finished, take yourself slowly back from the memory of the past to your present.

Every time you repeat this exercise, you will connect your mantra and ritual more powerfully to your flow state. Once you have this tool in your arsenal, you can use it in your pursuit of your Cool Impossible. Calling on your mantra and ritual while remembering that wellspring of positive feeling will distract you from your fears and remind you that they are just creations of your imagination. Once past your fears, you can refocus on your goal and present moment. You now have this ability to be exactly the way you want to be and act anytime you need it.

When things get tough, when you think the worst about yourself and want to give up on your dreams, reconnect to this flow state through the mantra and ritual. But do not even limit it to these "big" crossroads. If you need a boost during a race or workout, or just throughout your day, whether mentally or physically, this performance technique is there for you. All together: mantra, ritual, feeling. And you will be in a place to perform.

You are now ready to use visualization to help train your mind and prepare for day-to-day challenges and situations. You will likely use this visualization technique more than any other. I do. It's the key to creating the performance you want.

As an example, let's say you have an upcoming race. If it's a big event for you, I'd spend time each night for a week leading up to the event practicing this visualization technique. Get used to doing it, and getting it just right. That said, you can do this type of visualization anytime, sometimes minutes before the challenge. Whenever you need to perform at something.

Here, let me walk you through a practice you might do each night before a race. Close your eyes; take yourself through your mind's pathways again to the race in the future. Begin with the evening before. See yourself eating a good meal and readying for bed. See yourself easing into a peaceful slumber. Go for detail, as much of it as you can. See yourself wake up on the morning of the race. What time does the clock say? Feel yourself rising from bed with energy and calm, a warm, radiant feeling of health. See yourself eating your prerace meal; sense exactly what you would like to feel that morning: a little anxiousness and nerves. Smile and say to yourself, "Perfect."

Now you're dressing for the race, putting on your shorts, your jersey, your shoes, tying those laces tight. See yourself warm up; feel the deep breaths of air in your lungs that wake up your muscles. Create everything exactly the way you want it to go and feel. See yourself at the start, jumping up and down to stay warm. Hear the crack of the gun. Feel your body moving for the first time, running strong, fast, sure. See yourself at every step of the race. Imagine a low point, that moment when the legs feel weak, your breathing is hard, and you want to slow down, quit even—then see how you respond, how you stop those negative thoughts, how you use your mantra and ritual to find your flow and forge ahead, better, stronger than before. Take yourself through every part of the race, making it as real as you can. You hear the cheers of the crowd. You see the finish and your time on the clock. You feel yourself breaking across the finish line, achieving the result you wanted, arms high, a smile spread across your face. Feel that success. See your success. Create your success.

Now open your eyes. You're ready. Your body and your mind are now trained on the day ahead and can find this groove that you've visualized and follow it.

And if you feel like you got stuck during your visualization on a certain point or two, go back; do it again. This is expected. In a way you're watching a movie of the event ahead. Sometimes you have to hit pause, slow it down, speed it up to see and find all the details. But keep at it and trust that you'll become better at this visualization. Once you've seen its power, you will come back to it again and again.

On to the big visualization, your Cool Impossible. From the day you create your big ambition, to the weeks, months, years even, that you need to realize it, keep coming back to seeing it happening in your mind's eye. Visualize everything about your goal. See yourself preparing for it. See yourself making the journey, every step of the way. Allow your mind to drift in all directions around your Cool Impossible. Put yourself right into that day when you accomplish it. Know exactly when you will accomplish it. Feel that glory. Then come back; come back to the present. Open your eyes. Know one thing above all else: Your Cool Impossible is there for you every step of the way.

ATHLETICISM = AWARENESS

Almost back to the trailhead. Hear that babbling stream? A beautiful sound, right? There's that fallen tree we used to cross over the water on our way up. Watch your step on the way down; always look where you want to go, not where you don't—no need to take a cold splash now, though you're probably thinking it might be refreshing. That was a fast descent. Another good run.

Awareness. Everywhere—from the philosophy to the methods of training your mind—awareness is the central issue. Be aware of your thoughts, your fears, so you can focus on achieving your goals.

Be aware of the influence of your past, both good and bad. Be aware of the voices in your head to keep them from leading you astray. Be aware of the future, what you want from it, in it. Be aware of when you need to call on your mantras and rituals. Be aware of what you see and are able to create in your mind's eye. Be aware so you can be in the flow and so the world opens itself up to every possibility, athletic or otherwise. The only thing impossible is failure.

9

THE COOL IMPOSSIBLE

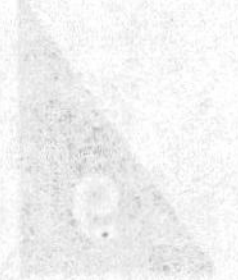

YOUR SEVENTH AND last day in Jackson Hole. This week's flown by. Lots to take in, I know. Hope it's been fun for you. I hope you see a path forward now with your running, maybe in other parts of your life as well.

Before you leave, one more run. Take it as you feel. We drive back into Grand Teton National Park and turn down a gravel road through a sagebrush meadow. Those shrubs, once dried out and uprooted, are tumbleweeds, like the ones you see in old Westerns, drifting across Main Street before the big gunfight. Yes, they're real.

We roll into a small lot by the Lupine Meadows Trailhead. That monster jagged peak straight ahead . . . that's the Grand Teton, 13,770 feet high. This is the trail that climbers take to reach the summit. Some even do the ascent in a day. I mean, it's possible—three hours possible, if you sprint most of the way up the seven thousand feet of vertical. The air's pretty thin up top. However, most do it in a two-day journey. They sleep overnight on the saddle separating the Middle Teton and the Grand, then climb to the peak the next day.

We've started early enough to make it all the way, if you want. Don't give me a look. All I'm saying is, it's possible.

And easier now than later, because the Tetons are still growing. Every hundred years we're talking another one inch or so in height as the tectonic plates underneath our feet collide, one downward, one up. There's a metaphor in there somewhere about great heights beginning at the base, but I'll leave that for you to decipher.

Onward. We run down the trail into the trees. What if we come upon another bear, a bigger one than a cub? you ask. I forgot the bear spray, but brought the camera. I'll take pictures. Ha, ha! you say.

We cross a bridge. Hold up. On the opposite side is a little surprise: Margot. Don't be fooled by her looks. In her late forties, that slight birdlike mother of five with wispy blond hair and a pretty face is an Ironman triathlete who's qualified for several world-championship competitions. As you'll see when we head up the trail together, she's true iron inside.

Since I've done all the teaching over the past week, I thought you'd like a little change, maybe to meet someone who's come through the other side of my training. As always, let's talk and run. These first few miles are gentle enough for that.

Margot tells you about herself first. In St. Louis, soon after she had her fifth child, she took to running to relieve some postpartum depression. Pretty soon she was training for her first triathlon. She just had that competitive spirit. Then Margot and her family moved out to Idaho. A big move to a small town. A change in life, a change in style. An adventure.

She continued to run, but with increasing pain, particularly on trails. She met me, but was soon after crippled by injury. Basically the ligaments in her right ankle had torn away due to an old college sport injury. Surgery followed. She wasn't sure whether she would even run again, let alone compete.

"I wanted to try, so I put myself in Eric's hands completely," Margot tells you. Before the surgery, she had taken some of my coaching, but still used orthotics and big shoes and trained by following a schedule she had bought from some guy working in a running store back in St. Louis.

After surgery, she started from nothing, hobbling on crutches. "We began with foot strength, doing the slant board work, slow, patient. Eric loves his slant board." The recovery boot would come off before the workout, then go back on afterward. When she took her first run several months later wearing minimal shoes, she felt stability in her foot like never before. It was the first of several breakthrough moments.

"Then Eric and I worked on my form at the track, eliminating my habit of overstriding, which I didn't even know I had."

Her running efficiency increased. Then came the strategic running foundation.

"I didn't like the heart rate monitor at first," she says. "I used to just go out for runs."

Though the program was hard and took a lot of discipline, the zones and diversity of workouts in the program became fun. She felt herself getting stronger, faster, and this allowed her to run longer, better than she had ever before in her life.

"You wouldn't see it every day," she tells you. "But over time, the improvements are unmistakable."

The slopes are beginning to steepen quite a bit. You're feeling it in your legs, in your lungs. This is getting hard, but Margot effortlessly keeps talking from behind you, urging you forward.

"Then all of sudden, things come together, and I had a breakthrough workout, accomplishing a distance I'd never done with such speed and ease. It's like I was running on air, everything feeling so good. Have faith; that will happen for you too."

The nutrition, she tells you, the twenty-day detox. That was not easy.

"I'm a self-admitted sugar addict, a work in progress," she says, but now she's much more aware of what she eats, and that helps in itself.

Then she speaks of awareness, of training her mind. This came during the physical work. "I had no awareness at first. Zero. But now I am very aware." One of her three-word mantras was, "Relax. Perform. Persist." Whenever she felt herself mentally waning, questioning whether she could continue on with a training run or strength exercise, she repeated her mantra, ritual, feeling. And *boom*: "The negative side was turned off and I was in the flow."

Margot tells you that eight months after her surgery, she ran a triathlon and qualified for the world championships. You turn, not quite believing her. She has a big smile on her face. She's telling the truth. Since then, she's continued to compete at a high level. But now she's thinking of veering off from racing. She wants to take her athleticism, her strength, on new adventures. She wants to run the Rim-to-Rim-to-Rim in the Grand Canyon. And she wants to ascend the Grand Teton. That's her new Cool Impossible, and she's out here today training for exactly that.

"Good luck with your own," she says, then waves, and she takes a split in the trail toward Surprise Lake. So strong, so fast—Margot is gone, lost amid the trees before you can thank her.

I hope you got something from meeting Margot. Now, you and me, we're heading up to Garnet Canyon, the way to the Grand Teton. You slow down to a walk. The air is thinning. You've already ascended two thousand feet of vertical, more than half at a run. Well-done. Maybe you'll want to run some more ahead, but for now, we'll hike up as far as you want to take it.

We take several switchbacks, giving us a perfect view of Taggart Lake at the base of the canyon. There's another bugle call of an elk. It's mating season somewhere in the trees below. An hour later, we head into Garnet Canyon at ten thousand feet of elevation. South Teton looms up to our left. The steep cliff wall to the right . . . that's part of Grand Teton, but given our angle, it's blocking our view of the peak. No worries. It's there, waiting to be reached when you're ready to reach it. For now, we're on this stretch of the climb, the trail littered with small round stones fallen from the mountainside. Stay in the flow.

Here's where I want to give you the big speech, the one right before you take this trail to wherever you want it to take you. I can't promise you grandiloquence, but know at least that I mean what I say, believe it in every fiber of my being. I try to live my words as best as I can in my own life.

Climb up onto this boulder with me; here, grab my hand—I'll pull you up. Take a seat. Notice how quiet it is. Seems so at first, but then come the sounds—all natural: the stream running over the rocks, the wind, the birds, the rumble of a storm in the far distance. But you don't notice these unless you're aware. The mountains are freedom. They don't care what kind of runner you are: an ultramarathoner, a champion 10K'er, or just starting. We are all the same up here. The mountain doesn't care how far you get.

Every step of the way up to this point, the three thousand feet of vertical, was beautiful—and constantly changing. Two miles down, you thought the lakes were too stunning for words. Then you took a switchback and they were gone, but another view, one of the canyon in the brilliant sunshine, opened itself up to you. Another switchback. Then the peak of Middle Teton framed in a scattering of clouds. New views. New perspectives. The way down will be the same.

I want you to remember this day. Notice how free you feel right now, how everything is so big, expansive, open. Notice how everything feels possible, within your grasp. Whenever you need it, this feeling can be with you. Embrace it. Tuck this feeling inside your pack and take it with you everywhere you go. When you create your Cool Impossible, this is how I want you to feel. Visualize this day and draw on this feeling.

As we sit here, I want you to start to understand how amazing it is to just know you have this ability to live freely and create anything you want for the future. In the creating comes the sizzle, the buzz, the happiness. See how fun and insanely brilliant it is to think beyond your wildest dreams. This is what the Cool Impossible is about: creating this experience and just going with it. Every day, every run, you can feel this way when you have this memory of the mountain with you. It's this feeling right now, this unbelievable feeling that you can do anything.

In this freedom, our mind explores without inhibitions, without judgments. See what I mean? I can see it on your face. You feel almost embarrassed to be feeling this way, but go for it. Go ahead; create that fantasy. Have fun; make it a game to create the unbelievable. That is what living is about. Climb on, I say.

Failure is not possible right now. I can see you almost smirking because you are starting to have crazy-good creative thoughts. Go with it; see where they take you. I have been your guide; now let the mountain guide you. Trust where your mind takes you; it will not lead you astray. There are no thoughts up here in the mountain, just endless impossibles to be explored. The trail will no doubt change along the way, rocky, smooth, winding, steep—bring it on. After all, fears are necessary and tell us we're on the right path.

When you know your fears will come, notice how that lessens their impact. You have the choice to move past them. Notice how strong this makes you feel. You no longer need confidence, because you have awareness. You no longer need more ability, because you now have the choice to be an athlete. After all, it is just a choice, and you now have it—which is all we need up here in the mountains. You have the choice to be exactly the type of runner and person you want to be. No matter where you live, no matter what job you do, no matter what your running experience, daydream the impossible; embrace the discipline required to go after it and try it.

But here's the truth, as I see it: Realizing your Cool Impossible is great. If you succeed, fantastic. Place the trophy on your shelf, mount the medal, put your picture crossing the finish line in a frame. But achieving that goal is not what will make you happy. Well, not enduringly happy. You'll feel a momentary triumph, but then it'll be gone. I can't tell you how many ultramarathoners I've coached who found themselves depressed after finishing their first fifty-miler. Do you know why?

It's the climbing that makes you happy, the one where you work the plan day after day, sticking to your discipline. Concentrating on form, doing those stability disk exercises, getting up and running your scheduled run, skipping that dessert, focusing on your present fears and disarming them, dispelling thoughts of success or failure and living in the present, here and now and in the flow—that's the joy. Once you experience that, once you're aware of how much happiness you draw from the climbing, you'll want it more and more.

Pretty soon, you'll achieve one Cool Impossible and want to follow it with another cooler, more impossible ambition simply to get that feeling back. You'll let go of "Can I do it?" and replace it with "Can I do it today?"—and the answer is yes. Like Margot, you'll "do what's required." Yes, because of discipline—discipline is the ultimate performance, but also the ultimate freedom because of the intoxicating joy of it all.

I quiet down. The speech is over. Together we scramble over a stretch of huge boulders, climbing up and down, the rocks secured together in a massive jigsaw puzzle. On the other side the trail resumes, now winding its way up toward a ridgeline under the shadow of Middle Teton.

Instead of continuing forward, I bend down and take a drink from the rushing mountain stream to our left. I drink long and deep from the cool, fresh water. You follow me one more time and do the same.

Then I stand, clap my hand on your shoulder, and say, "Go ahead now, onward without me."

Maybe you're a little reluctant to go, maybe a little eager. Maybe both. But you go, embarking on your own, pursuing your own Cool Impossible, whether to the top of Grand Teton or beyond. Demand the impossible, I say. Have fun. Be in the flow.

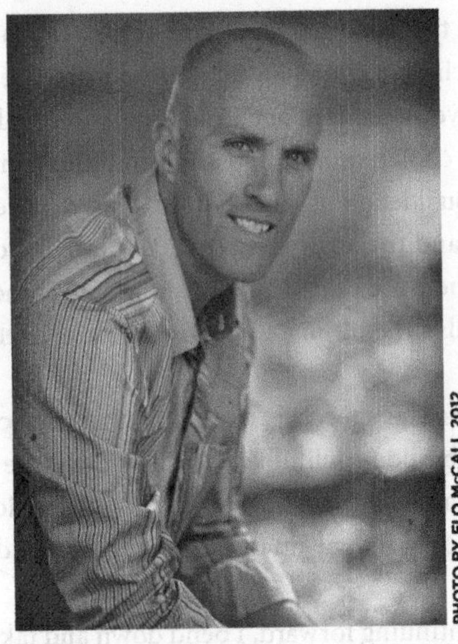

ERIC ORTON's experiences with the Tarahumara and his study of running, human performance, strength, and conditioning have led him to the cutting edge of the sport and made him the go-to guy for athletes everywhere. Christopher McDougall is just one of the coach's many success stories. The former fitness director for the University of Colorado Health Sciences Center, Orton now personally oversees the training of dozens of athletes, from recreational racers to elite ultramarathoners.

CONNECT ONLINE

thecoolimpossible.com

twitter.com/borntoruncoach